Synthesis Lectures on Technology and Health

Series Editors

Ron Baecker, University of Toronto, Toronto, Canada

Andrew Sixsmith, Simon Fraser University, Vancouver, Canada

Sumi Helal, University of Florida, Gainesville, USA

Gillian R. Hayes, University of California, Irvine, USA

The series publishes state-of-the-art short books on transformative technologies for health, wellness, and independent living. Our scope of publishing in the expanding health tech field includes:

- Technology in support of active and healthy living and aging
- Digital technologies for health- and social-care improvement
- Diagnostic, screening, and tracking tools
- Assistive and rehabilitative technologies

The series includes a subseries of books published in partnership with Canada's AGE-WELL that specifically addresses their 8 AgeTech Challenge Areas. Each lecture introduces the context in which the technology is used—wellness, health, medicine, special needs, or other contexts. Authors present and explain the technology and review promising applications and opportunities as well as limitations and challenges. They include material on their own work while surveying the broader landscape of related research, development, and impact.

Arlene Astell · David Clayton

AgeTech for Staying Connected

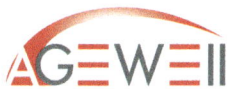

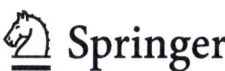

Arlene Astell
University of Toronto
Toronto, ON, Canada

Northumbria University
Newcastle upon Tyne, UK

David Clayton
University of Leicester
Leicester, UK

ISSN 2771-7054 ISSN 2771-7070 (electronic)
Synthesis Lectures on Technology and Health
ISBN 978-3-031-87030-9 ISBN 978-3-031-87031-6 (eBook)
https://doi.org/10.1007/978-3-031-87031-6

© The Editor(s) (if applicable) and The Author(s), under exclusive license to Springer Nature Switzerland AG 2026

This work is subject to copyright. All rights are solely and exclusively licensed by the Publisher, whether the whole or part of the material is concerned, specifically the rights of translation, reprinting, reuse of illustrations, recitation, broadcasting, reproduction on microfilms or in any other physical way, and transmission or information storage and retrieval, electronic adaptation, computer software, or by similar or dissimilar methodology now known or hereafter developed.

The use of general descriptive names, registered names, trademarks, service marks, etc. in this publication does not imply, even in the absence of a specific statement, that such names are exempt from the relevant protective laws and regulations and therefore free for general use.

The publisher, the authors and the editors are safe to assume that the advice and information in this book are believed to be true and accurate at the date of publication. Neither the publisher nor the authors or the editors give a warranty, expressed or implied, with respect to the material contained herein or for any errors or omissions that may have been made. The publisher remains neutral with regard to jurisdictional claims in published maps and institutional affiliations.

This Springer imprint is published by the registered company Springer Nature Switzerland AG
The registered company address is: Gewerbestrasse 11, 6330 Cham, Switzerland

If disposing of this product, please recycle the paper.

Acknowledgements

The authors would like to thank the Science and Technology for Aging Research (STAR) Institute, of Simon Fraser University, for its administrative and financial support and AGE-WELL for its financial support.

The authors would particularly like to thank the AGE-WELL community—The Network Management Office, researchers, older adults and caregivers, and partners. Their passion for innovation was essential in developing and sustaining this book's creation. Thank you for your collaborative spirit.

The authors would also like to thank The Centre for Assistive Technology and Connected Healthcare (CATCH), University of Sheffield for their permission to use photographs taken during the Technology for Healthy Ageing and Well-being Project (THAW). For further details visit https://catch.sites.sheffield.ac.uk/projects/technology-for-healthy-ageing-and-wellbeing-thaw.

Photographs used in this publication are also from The Centre for Ageing Better, Age-Positive Image Library. For further details visit https://ageingbetter.resourcespace.com/pages/search.php.

AGE-WELL (www.agewell-nce.ca) is Canada's Technology and Aging Network. The pan-Canadian network brings together researchers, older adults, caregivers, partner organizations, and future leaders to accelerate the delivery of technology-based solutions that make a meaningful difference in the lives of Canadians. AGE-WELL researchers are producing technologies, services, policies, and practices that improve quality of life for older adults and caregivers, and generate social and economic benefits for Canada. AGE-WELL's work is supported through Government of Canada funding programs.

The STAR (Science and Technology for Aging Research) Institute (www.sfu.ca/starinstitute) at Simon Fraser University (SFU) is committed to supporting community-engaged research in the rapidly growing area of technology and aging. The Institute supports the development and implementation of technologies to address many of the health challenges encountered in old age, as well as addresses the social, commercial, and policy aspects of using and accessing technologies. STAR also supports the AGE-WELL network.

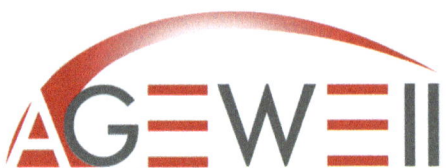
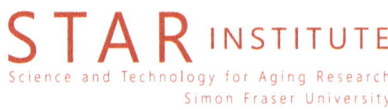

Contents

1 Introduction 1
   1.1 Staying Connected with AgeTech 1
        1.1.1 Staying Connected is Essential to Well-Being 2
        1.1.2 AGE-WELL Challenge Areas 3
   1.2 This Book 4
        1.2.1 Who is This Book for? 5
        1.2.2 Organization of the Book 6
   References 7

2 The Importance of Staying Connected 9
   2.1 The Challenge 9
   2.2 Persona and Scenario: Mrs. Adeniyi 10
   2.3 Loneliness and Social Isolation 11
   2.4 Physical and Mental Health 12
   References 15

3 AgeTech for Staying Connected 19
   3.1 The Challenge 20
   3.2 Persona and Scenario: Wen 20
   3.3 Types of AgeTech for Staying Connected 22
        3.3.1 Internet 22
        3.3.2 Videoconferencing 22
        3.3.3 Conversational Agents 22
        3.3.4 Robots 23
        3.3.5 Virtual Reality 24
        3.3.6 Mixed Reality Technologies 26
   3.4 Key Initiative #VoiceforLoneliness 26
   References 26

4	**Supporting Social Interaction with Existing Social Networks**		29
	4.1	The Challenge	30
	4.2	What's in This Chapter?	30
	4.3	Persona and Scenario: Maria	30
	4.4	Technology Solutions	32
		4.4.1 Remote and Virtual Connections	32
		4.4.2 Social Media	34
		4.4.3 Digital Storytelling	34
	4.5	Key Initiative—Teledining	35
	4.6	Find Out More	37
	References		37
5	**Social Isolation and Mental Well-Being**		39
	5.1	The Challenge	40
	5.2	What's in This Chapter?	41
	5.3	Persona and Scenario: Simon	41
	5.4	Mental Health	42
	5.5	Technology Solutions	43
		5.5.1 Mood Apps	43
		5.5.2 Technology for Social Isolation	43
		5.5.3 Chatbots	45
	5.6	Key Initiative—OnHand	46
	5.7	Find Out More	46
	References		47
6	**Staying Connected to Recreation and Leisure**		49
	6.1	The Challenge	50
	6.2	What's in This Chapter?	50
	6.3	Persona and Scenario: Mathilde	50
	6.4	Technology for Recreation and Leisure	52
		6.4.1 Museums and Art Galleries	52
		6.4.2 Digital Games	53
		6.4.3 Making Music	55
		6.4.4 Singing	56
	6.5	Key Initiative—Art on the Brain	58
	6.6	Find Out More	59
	References		59
7	**Staying Connected for Cognitive Stimulation**		61
	7.1	The Challenge	62
		7.1.1 Social Connectedness and Dementia	62
		7.1.2 Social Interventions for Cognition	62

	7.2	What's in This Chapter?	64
	7.3	Persona and Scenario: Grace	64
	7.4	Technology for Social Connection and Cognitive Stimulation	65
		7.4.1 Playing Games for Cognitive Stimulation	65
		7.4.2 Group Activities	66
	7.5	Key Initiative—Dancing to Improve Health and Stay Connected	69
	7.6	Find Out More	71
		References	71
8	**Staying Connected for Intimacy**	75
	8.1	The Challenge	76
	8.2	What's in This Chapter?	77
	8.3	Persona and Scenario: Edwin	77
	8.4	Technology for Intimacy	78
		8.4.1 Hugging Technology	78
		8.4.2 Online Relationships	79
		8.4.3 Technology for Sexual Activity	81
	8.5	Key Initiative—Lovotics	84
	8.6	Find Out More	84
		References	85
9	**Staying Connected to Healthcare**	87
	9.1	The Challenge	88
	9.2	What's in This Chapter?	88
	9.3	Persona and Scenario: Mei	88
	9.4	Technology for Connecting to Healthcare	89
		9.4.1 Self-management Tools	89
		9.4.2 Telehealth/Telemedicine	90
		9.4.3 Online Resources	91
		9.4.4 Chatbots	94
	9.5	Key Initiative—Keeping Indigenous Older People Connected to Healthcare	95
	9.6	Find Out More	95
		References	96
10	**Staying Connected and the Digital Divide**	99
	10.1	The Challenge	100
	10.2	What's in This Chapter?	100
	10.3	Persona and Scenario: Roxanne	100
	10.4	Understanding Digital Exclusion and the Digital Divide	102
		10.4.1 Getting Access to the Internet When on Low Income	104
		10.4.2 Accessibility and Usability of Equipment	105
		10.4.3 Motivation, Support, and the 'Digitally Dismissive'	106

	10.5	Meeting the Exclusion Challenge	106
		10.5.1 Addressing Data Poverty (Access to the Internet)	106
		10.5.2 Addressing Device Poverty (Access to Equipment)	107
		10.5.3 Addressing Skills Poverty (The Ability to Use Technology Safely and with Confidence)	108
	10.6	Not Just Assistive Technology	109
	10.7	The Technology Pipeline and Need for Co-creation, Co-design, and Co-production	110
	References		111
11	**Emerging Issues and Future Directions**		113
	11.1	The Challenge	114
	11.2	What's in This Chapter?	114
	11.3	Older Age and Societal Change	114
	11.4	Ethically Incorporating Technology into Services	115
		11.4.1 Spotlight Issue—Telehealth for Delivering Bad News	115
		11.4.2 Face-to-Face Versus Remote Contact	116
	11.5	Persona and Scenario: Mr. Emeka	118
		11.5.1 Spotlight on Community Initiatives: Men in Sheds	119
	11.6	A Personalised Approach to Addressing Social Isolation and Loneliness	120
		11.6.1 Focus on Individuals Who Need Support the Most	121
		11.6.2 Focus on Individual Outcomes with AgeTech	121
	References		122
12	**Conclusion**		125
	References		127

Introduction

1

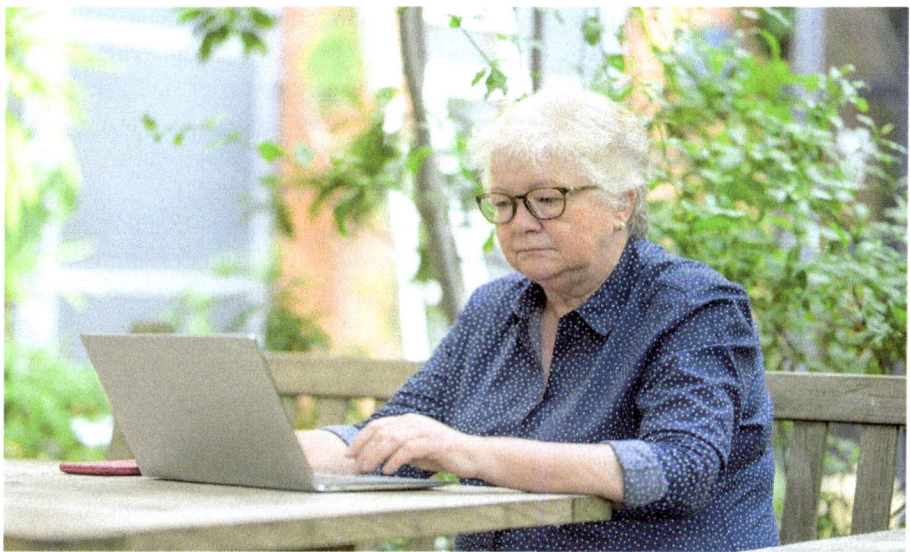

Image 1.1 *Credit* David Tett/Ageing Better

1.1 Staying Connected with AgeTech

Humans are social beings who are born ready to connect with others. Throughout our lives we are sustained by our connections with other people: our relationships with family and friends, lovers and colleagues, teammates and classmates, communities and societies all define who we are and shape our sense of self. Cut off from others we experience loneliness and social isolation that can lead to depression, poor health and increased risk of cognitive impairment or death.

Multiple personal, social, and economic reasons make staying connected essential for living and aging well. On an individual level, our mental health and well-being are strongly influenced by our relationships and connectedness with other people. People need to feel connected to others and in the presence of those who they like, trust and can be together with (Cacioppo & Patrick, 2008). Socially, close relationships contribute to our identity and place in the world—they confirm our roles such as partner, parent, friend, or colleague. Feeling connected, having people to interact with, and opportunities to do so contribute to our feeling of being in the social world. As we age various factors, such as loss of close family and friends, family living further away, reduced opportunities to make new relationships, and declining health or mobility may all contribute to fewer and less frequent social interactions.

Technology offers many ways for people to stay connected and can be particularly useful for older adults (Image 1.1). AgeTech is a recent term for technologies that benefit older adults. However, this term is not universally accepted, with critics arguing that designing exclusively for older adults lacks inclusivity in design and risks perpetuating ageist stereotypes (Briscoll & Carroll, 2021). Advocates propose that AgeTech encapsulates a holistic approach to the needs and wants of older adults that will produce technologies to enhance increasing life expectancy (Rubeis et al., 2022).

Within this book series, AgeTech is applied broadly to the range of technologies being created or leveraged to empower individuals in their later lives. In the realm of staying connected, this includes information and communication technologies (ICTs), robotics, mobile technologies, artificial intelligence (AI), augmented reality (AR) and virtual reality (VR), and smart home systems. The wide range of current and emerging AgeTech offers great potential to meet growing global demands for keeping people connected as they age, reduce loneliness and social isolation and improve their well-being. However, AgeTech can also present challenges and the potential to disadvantage and exclude older people further if they lack the resources and right support to access AgeTech. This book aims to present examples of AgeTech research and innovation alongside the challenges that need to be tackled to empower older adults to stay connected.

1.1.1 Staying Connected is Essential to Well-Being

Loneliness and social isolation are linked with poor mental health, an issue which was highlighted by the COVID-19 pandemic. Loneliness and social isolation are also linked to physical health and morbidity as well as increasing the risk of cognitive decline associated with dementia. Loneliness has specifically been associated with an increased risk of mortality (Perissinotto et al., 2012), with some estimates suggesting the impact on mortality is comparable to smoking and alcohol consumption (Holt-Lunstad et al., 2010).

Connected communities provide support for their members but also activities and opportunities for social participation. Reducing risks associated with being disconnected, by keeping people in touch with family, friends and communities and making new connections, can reduce demands on healthcare and other services. As the global population ages, concerted efforts are needed to share best practices and promote social connections in later life.

Another way that staying connected can be understood as an essential aspect of later life is the rise in digital delivery of services and resources that older people need or wish to access. Shopping, banking, and healthcare are examples of activities and services that are moving more and more online. This book was written during and after the COVID-19 pandemic, which has seen an accelerated process of remote access and delivery. The pandemic presented an imperative for Staying Connected remotely, e.g., clinical consultations; this required older people to have reliable access to devices and the Internet, as well as in many cases learning to use new applications, e.g., one or more video-conferencing platforms.

Acquiring devices and internet access requires support plus training to use them effectively. Many organizations that work with older adults have pivoted to provide online services and support to their members or customers to access them. Across the world, multiple initiatives have sprung up to bring technology to older people and connect them to support networks and vital services. However, a divide still exists between those who can realise the benefits of using AgeTech and those who cannot because of barriers to access and use.

1.1.2 AGE-WELL Challenge Areas

It is within this context that staying connected remains a challenge for AgeTech. The rise of remote interaction and provision perfectly illustrates the AGE-WELL concept of a Challenge Area. As part of AGE-WELL's national consultation into *'The Future of Technology and Aging Research in Canada'* (2018), people across Canada identified staying connected as one of eight major Challenge Areas for living well in later life (see Table 1.1).

AGE-WELL Challenge Areas are *"important but difficult and complex problem areas that demand innovation and deployment of real-world solutions."* In this context, a challenge is NOT just about problems, i.e., areas of lack or need or gaps in provision. Nor is a Challenge Area just about a topic for focusing research activity and resources. AGE-WELL Challenge Areas are priorities for living and aging well that (i) require research and innovation, (ii) present economic opportunities and (iii) have the potential for making a positive contribution to Canadian society and government policy. Whilst initiated in Canada, these Challenge Areas have global relevance for social connection as illustrated by the international examples of AgeTech and personas in this book.

Table 1.1 AGE-WELL challenge areas[1]

1	Supportive homes & communities
2	Health care & health service delivery
3	Autonomy & independence
4	Cognitive health & dementia
5	Mobility & transportation
6	Healthy lifestyles & wellness
7	Staying connected
8	Financial wellness & employment

1.2 This Book

This book aims to provide insights and inspiration for everyone interested in promoting social connectedness for older adults. It combines current research into AgeTech for Staying Connected with personas from around the world illustrating common circumstances and situations that can lead to older people becoming disconnected, lonely, or isolated. With contributions from Canada, Europe, Latin America, Asia and Africa, these personas highlight some of the factors that are common across countries, as well as others that may require adjustments for cultural differences. Forthcoming publications in this series will focus on healthy aging which will also highlight issues of social isolation and its impact on mental and cognitive health.

Illustrated with examples from the AGE-WELL network plus innovators across the world, including service providers, cultural and heritage organizations, charitable and community groups, this book—AgeTech for Staying Connected—will provide readers with an accessible resource for understanding the range and sample applications of existing and emerging technologies for social connection. While not intended to be exhaustive,

---

[1] These eight AGE-WELL Challenge Areas resulted from an extensive review and public consultation process carried out across the AGE-WELL Network with its members, partners, older Canadians, and caregivers. Additionally, a review of Canadian provincial and territorial policy priorities relating to older adults was conducted by Advancing Policies and Practices in Technology and Aging (APPTA), the New Brunswick-based AGE-WELL National Innovation Hub. An environmental scan of national and international policy documents was also carried out by the STAR Institute at Simon Fraser University. From these extensive activities a short list of 18 Challenge Areas was produced. These were then used as the basis of five local consultations held across Canada in Vancouver, Edmonton, Winnipeg, Toronto, and Montreal in 2018. Members of AGE-WELL's International Scientific Advisory Committee also provided their perspectives on this short list. Finally, feedback gathered from over 1,000 stakeholders who participated in the in-person consultations or completed an online survey open to the general public, was used to prioritize the final set of eight Challenge Areas—more information can be found here:

https://agewell-nce.ca/wp-content/uploads/2018/05/Booklet_8_Challenges_English_2019oct2_digital.pdf

1.2 This Book 5

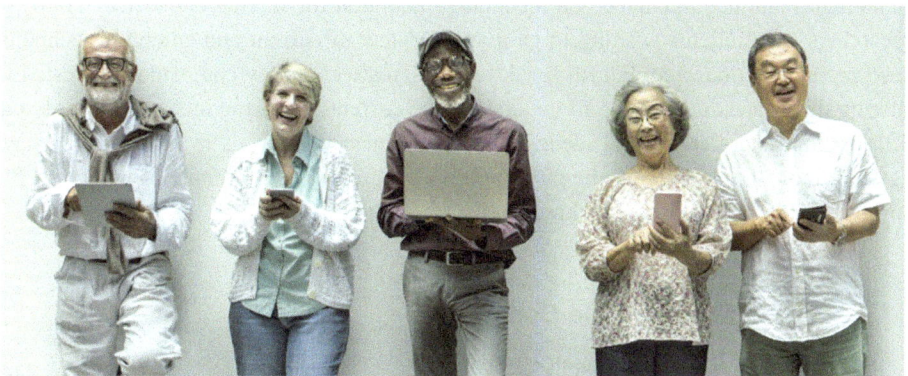

Image 1.2 *Credit* Shutterstock: Rawpixel.com

this book will cover some basic information on common obstacles and barriers to technology development and adoption, things to keep in mind when using technology, and making the most of what is available. Examples of digital tools, services, and resources are provided because of the need for an accessible guide to help people understand what is currently available, how it can be accessed and where new technologies are emerging to support social connection.

The rise of commercial products, such as smartphones, tablets, and voice assistants, has highlighted the need for accessible information and guidance to help people seeking to engage with technologies. Once identified, people also need guidance and support on how to incorporate them into their lives and make the most of the available apps and services for staying connected. This book also highlights the challenges older people may face with AgeTech and the need for technology to be inclusive and person-centred. It is within this context that policy is required to address any barriers older people may face to realising the benefits of staying connected using AgeTech (Image 1.2).

1.2.1 Who is This Book for?

This book is aimed primarily at people looking to understand what developments have been made and are currently underway, what evidence exists for current technologies, and a summary of what sorts of AgeTech are available. The rapid pace of development, particularly with commercially available technologies, along with the competing claims being made for the benefits of many items, means that practical guidance is needed for people outside the fields of research and industry. It is hoped that this book will be helpful for a range of interested parties. First for older adults who wish to know more about what AgeTech is currently available that can assist them in staying connected. Second for organizations that provide services to older adults and are seeking to purchase or invest in technologies and need guidance on technology adoption for staying connected. Third for researchers and students wishing to gain an overview of current and emerging technologies for staying connected. Fourth for developers and technology companies interested in entering this space and looking to understand the current landscape in staying connected. Fifth, policymakers seeking to identify the emerging opportunities in AgeTech for staying connected and addressing the challenges of supporting older people to overcome the barriers of using these digital technologies.

1.2.2 Organization of the Book

This book is intended to serve as a brief introductory guide to the role of AgeTech in staying connected in later life. There are two introductory chapters followed by six chapters targeting different aspects of staying connected in later life. Specifically, Chapter 2 examines the importance of staying connected in terms of individual health and wellbeing. Chapter 3 introduces the main areas where AgeTech is being developed for staying connected. Chapters 4–9 address six different aspects of life where people may benefit from AgeTech to stay connected: Chapter 4 addresses maintaining social interaction with existing networks; Chapter 5 looks at tackling social isolation; Chapter 6 examines opportunities for staying connected to recreation and leisure; Chapter 7 looks at the importance of staying connected for cognitive stimulation; Chapter 8 explores our need for intimacy; Chapter 9 examines different ways AgeTech can help us stay connected to healthcare. These chapters include common factors that may lead people to become disconnected from family, friends, and wider society such as ill health, bereavement, and loss of confidence. Chapter 10 examines the barriers to accessibility and availability of AgeTech for staying connected and the challenge for policymakers in addressing the digital divide. Chapter 11 looks at emerging issues and future directions in AgeTech for staying connected. Finally, Chapter 12 sums up the topics covered in a conclusion. Chapters 2–11 are each illustrated by a persona and scenario that relates to the specific chapter topic, followed by examples of existing and emerging AgeTech for the specific issue, e.g., staying connected for intimacy. We are extremely grateful to the authors who are experts in staying connected in their fields or countries, and who have composed these especially for this book.

After reading this book, the reader should:

- Understand the importance of staying connected in later life.
- Appreciate the potential of technology-based products and services to empower people to stay connected.
- Have a better sense of the main directions for research and innovation for staying connected.
- Identify how research can translate into real-world products and services.

- Develop an awareness of key AgeTech products, services, and initiatives for staying connected.
- Understand some of the key policy and ethical challenges relating to AgeTech for staying connected.

References

AGE-WELL. (2018). The Future of Technology and Aging Research in Canada. Available at https://agewell-nce.ca/wp-content/uploads/2019/01/Booklet_8_Challenges_English_5_final_PROOF_rev.pdf

Briscoe, G., & Carroll, S. (2021). Inclusive design: To AgeTech or not to AgeTech? Workshop. *International Federation on Ageing 2021*, Canada, pp. 9–12.

Cacioppo, J. T., & Patrick, W. (2008). *Loneliness: Human nature and the need for social connection.* WW Norton and Company.

Holt-Lunstad, J., Smith, T.B., & Layton, J. B. (2010). Social relationships and mortality risk: A meta-analytic review. *PLoS Med, 7*(7). https://doi.org/10.1371/journal.pmed.1000316

Perissinotto, C. M., Cenzer, I. S., & Covinsky, K. E. (2012). Loneliness in older persons: A predictor of functional decline and death. *Archives of Internal Medicine, 172*(14), 1078–1084.

Rubeis, G., Fang, M. L., & Sixsmith, A. (2022). Equity in AgeTech for ageing well in technology-driven places: The role of social determinants in designing AI-based assistive technologies. *Science and Engineering Ethics, 28*(6). https://doi.org/10.1007/s11948-022-00397-y

The Importance of Staying Connected 2

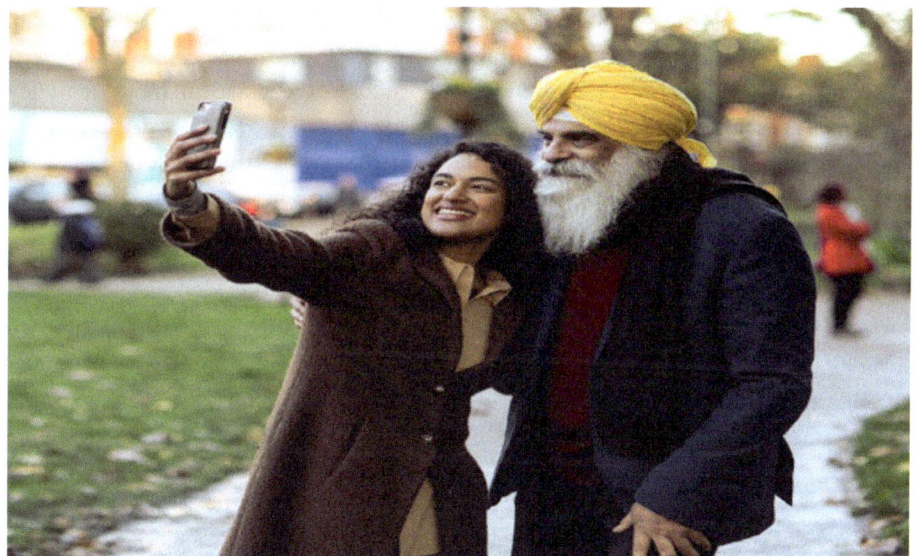

Image 2.1 *Credit* Peter Kindersley/ageing better

2.1 The Challenge

Humans are social beings. We come into the world equipped to connect with other people (Image 2.1). The cries of a newborn infant primarily serve a survival function to elicit a caregiver response (Bornstein et al., 2017). Over time, parents of newborns typically repeat and reinforce the sounds, facial expressions, and movements made by their infants.

These parent-infant interactions provide the foundation for a life of staying connected. Indeed, being connected to other people has been identified as one of three essential human needs. Self-determination theory (Ryan & Deci, 2000) identifies 'relatedness'— a sense of belonging and attachment to other people—as one of three *'psychological nutrients...essential for individuals' adjustment, integrity, and growth'* (Vansteenkiste et al., 2020, p. 1). Fulfilling our need for relatedness, along with 'autonomy' and 'competence' is vital for our health and well-being (Ryan & Deci, 2000). In later life, meeting our needs for relatedness, autonomy, and competence can become difficult for a variety of reasons, increasing the risk of older people becoming disconnected from family, friends, and society.

2.2 Persona and Scenario: Mrs. Adeniyi[1]

Persona: Mrs Adeniyi is a 74-year-old retired widow who lives in Ibadan, Nigeria. She has three male children, all living in different states far from Ibadan. Mrs Adeniyi lives alone, which is often not the case in Nigeria, as children and grandchildren often allow grandparents or parents to live in the same house. However, Mrs Adeniyi's children cannot afford to move her in with them because they are all employed in precarious jobs and merely survive with their respective families. As a retiree, she receives a 36,000 Naira (CAD$100) pension from the federal government, which is not consistent as she received her last pension in 2019, and she solely depends on her children for support and treatment costs.

Scenario: Mrs Adeniyi has lived with a diabetic foot ulcer for five years, limiting her mobility and preventing her from visiting friends and close family relations. She was only able to attend church services twice a week, which was very therapeutic for her. She uses the opportunity to engage and interact with her church members, who were her primary source of social support. Within the past year, Mrs Adeniyi has not attended church because her church building was relocated, preventing her from attending church again. She does not have any reliable source of transportation and cannot afford to pay 300 Naira (a little less than CAD$1) every week to attend church. One of her church members sometimes gave her a ride to church, but this was not consistent because the road to her house was in a very deplorable state. She tried to attend another church close to her home, but she did not feel that sense of belonging and, ever since, has stopped going to church. Just recently, her closest friend, who visited her every day, passed away. She feels so utterly alone, except when her children call her on the telephone, which happens once a week.

---

[1] Persona and scenario created by Blessing U. Ojembe BSc, MSc, Ph.D.(c); Michael E. Kalu, BMR.PT, MSc, Ph.D.(c); and Oyinlola Oluwagbemiga, BSW, MSW of McMaster University, Canada.

Her health condition (e.g., being diabetic) is a vital contributor to her being lonely. A geriatric social worker and physiotherapist currently manage her condition. The physiotherapist prescribed a scooter to enable her to move around in her neighbourhood. However, she cannot afford to get the scooter and even if she can afford it, there are associated factors that would limit its use. Among several factors, built environment barriers (no sidewalks for the scooters) and a transportation system (which is not age-friendly or accessible) will make it difficult for her to use the scooter. The physiotherapist later prescribed a walking aid—a tripod, but this walking aid can only enable her to move around in her home, limiting her ability to move beyond her home. The social worker advised her children to get her a television with access to cable channels, enabling her to know what is happening in Nigeria and to feel connected to the outside world. Also, her children are planning to relocate her close to one of them, ensuring that she does not continue to feel utterly abandoned and lonely.

2.3 Loneliness and Social Isolation

As we can see from the case of Mrs Adeniyi, multiple factors can contribute to an older person becoming lonely or isolated from their family and community. Older people are more likely to live alone, often through the death of a spouse or life partner, which coupled with mobility constraints, lack of motivation, lack of opportunities and lack of skills and access to information technologies, are among five barriers to older adults staying connected, that were identified by Baez et al. (2019). In the US, living alone coupled with declining participation in religious activities, led the former US Surgeon General to term this a 'loneliness epidemic' among the aging population (Murthy, 2017). Additionally, a decline in intergenerational households, is a major contributor to living alone, as successive generations of children move away for work (Ruggles, 2007). In the mid-19th Century, only 10% of older adults in the US lived alone, while 80% lived with family members, of which 70% were with children or children-in-law (Ruggles, 2001). In 2010 the number of older adults living with a child in the US had dropped to an estimated 19.4% (United Nations, 2017).

As demonstrated by Mrs Adeniyi's situation, changes in co-residence are not confined to Western countries. In 2017, the UN produced a report on the living arrangements of older adults across 143 countries for which data were available, covering 97% of those aged over 60 years old in 2010 (United Nations, 2017). This found that in Nigeria, where Mrs Adeniyi lives, 40% of older adults do not live with their children. However, across the world, the number of older adults living with their children varies widely. UN data from 121 countries found only 5.5% of older adults in the Netherlands lived with their children while in Afghanistan this was 94.8% (United Nations, 2017). Global trends indicated that in 73% of countries in Africa, 77% in Latin America and 93% in Asia, more than

50% of older adults live with their children but this was only the case in one European country—Albania (United Nations, 2017).

The terms *loneliness* and *social isolation* are often used interchangeably but they mean different things. Loneliness is the *subjective experience* of being alone whilst desiring to have interactions with other people (Perlman & Peplau, 1981). Social isolation, on the other hand, is an *objective state*…

> …in which the individual lacks a sense of belonging socially, lacks engagement with others, has a minimal number of social contacts and …[lack]…fulfilling and quality relationships (Nicholson, 2009, p. 1346).

Research suggests that loneliness affects at least one-third of older adults at some time but could reach almost 60% in some groups of older adults, such as those with severe health problems (Musich et al., 2015). This latter population includes 28% who report experiencing severe loneliness.

Loneliness is not confined to those who live alone in the community such as Mrs Adenyi. The UK Campaign to End Loneliness (2015) summarised the array of factors that contribute to loneliness in later life (Table 2.1). Identified as a risk factor for entering long-term care (Hanratty et al., 2018), high levels of loneliness have been reported among people who are living in care homes. This may seem surprising given care homes are multi-resident dwellings and people may be encouraged to move 'for the company'. However, Victor (2012) found 22–42% of residents reported severe loneliness compared to approximately 10% of community dwelling older adults. This may be compounded by visual impairment (Mann et al., 2020), hearing loss (Shukla et al., 2020) and frailty (Neves et al., 2019).

One impact of the COVID-19 pandemic was how the enforced isolation introduced to reduce the spread of the virus, heightened awareness of the importance of social interaction and the negative impact lack of interaction can have. One survey conducted in Ontario, Canada of people aged between 65 and 79 in the summer of 2020, found that in the previous week, 43% felt lonely some of the time including 8.3% who felt lonely always or often (Savage et al., 2021). The risk of loneliness was higher among women and those living alone. During the pandemic, multiple articles were reported on the impact of quarantine and social distancing measures on loneliness and isolation among older adults (e.g., Wu, 2020) and the negative effect of these on the physical and mental health of older adults (e.g., Sépulveda-Loyola et al., 2020).

2.4 Physical and Mental Health

In later life, loneliness and social isolation have been linked to both physical and mental health problems. A recent review found that loneliness presents a comparable risk for cardiovascular disease and early mortality to other well-established risk factors such as

2.4 Physical and Mental Health

Table 2.1 Risk factors for loneliness in later life (UK Campaign to End Loneliness, 2015)

Personal circumstances	Living alone
	Being single divorced, never married
	Living on a low income
	Living in residential care
Transitions	Bereavement
	Becoming a carer or giving up caring
	Retirement
Personal characteristics	Aged 75 plus
	From an ethnic minority community
	Being gay or lesbian
Health and disability	Poor health
	Immobility
	Cognitive impairment
	Sensory impairment
	Dual sensory impairment
Geography i.e., living in an area	With high levels of material deprivation
	In which crime is an issue

obesity or smoking (Paul et al., 2021). These authors proposed that the risk presented by loneliness might be indirect, mediated by a range of factors including poor health-related behaviour, such as smoking or lack of exercise, biological factors such as inflammation, or psychological factors such as depression. Loneliness has also been linked to functional decline including difficulty with activities of daily living (ADL), decline in mobility, or increased difficulty in stair climbing (Perissinotto et al., 2012). Additionally, a growing body of evidence confirms that loneliness increases mortality risk (e.g., Luo et al., 2012; Ward et al., 2021).

The lack of opportunities to interact with other people can result in poor mental health and well-being (Berg-Weger & Morley, 2020). Links with mental health have been long established, with work by Lowenthal (1964) almost 60 years ago directly relating social isolation to mental health problems in later life. Her illuminating article, examining a sample of 534 older adults admitted to the psychiatric screening wards of the San Francisco General Hospital in 1959, identified 52 individuals she classified as "pure' isolates'. These were defined as....

> People who had no friends or relatives involved in the decision-making process that led to hospitalization, and for whom no such persons could be located after they had been admitted to the psychiatric ward... no contact with a friend or relative in the two weeks prior to

admission… no contact of any kind with a friend or a relative for approximately three years (Lowenthal, 1964, p. 57).

Lowenthal also identified 56 'semi-isolates' who she described as individuals who had nobody involved in the decision-making but who did report some albeit casual social contacts in the period prior to admission (Image 2.2). Most individuals in both isolated subgroups were living alone before admission to the hospital. One case example illustrates the sorts of situations Lowenthal's isolated older adults were in:

> Mrs. C. is a 66-year-old retired nurse who has been a widow for 30 years. She went to the psychiatric ward voluntarily because she was "terribly nervous" and feared that she was developing an addiction to barbiturates she had taken since having a partial gastrectomy. Her diagnosis was psychogenic (affective disorder). She said she had no contact with relatives and that "all of my friends are gone." At another point in the interview, she said she had seen no one since her gastrectomy a year earlier. Still later, she remarked that she did not want her friends to know she is ill. At any rate, she refused to name friends, and at the second interview a year later, in a state hospital, she said she had spread the word that she was visiting her brother in British Columbia (Lowenthal, 1964, p. 57).

This case highlights several factors that are still pertinent today—loss of a spouse and close friends, not wanting others to know a person is ill, and putting others off

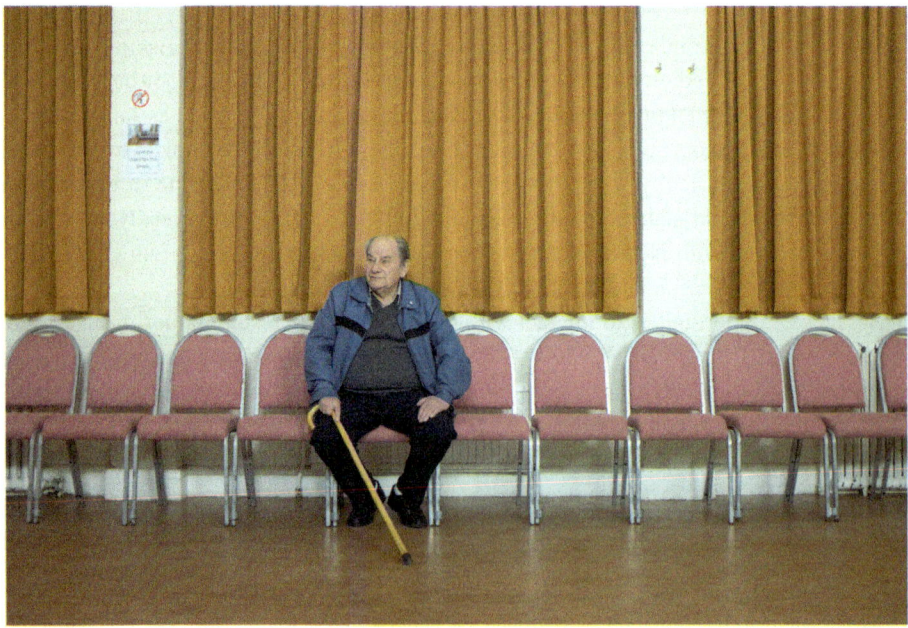

Image 2.2 *Credit* Mark Epstein/ageing better

(i.e., telling them she is visiting her brother) possibly to avoid having to discuss ill-health or how she feels. While there has been a shift to addressing more mental health issues in the community, the situations of Mrs C and others described by Lowenthal, are familiar today. For example, in a recent study discussing late-life mental health, older adults discussed their reluctance to burden others with their mental health issues and fear of the consequences of reporting them (e.g., being labelled, hospitalized, etc.) (Andrews et al., 2019).

Looking at specific mental illnesses, loneliness is linked to more depressive symptoms (Cacioppo et al., 2006) and greater symptom severity (Lee et al., 2021). In addition, an increased prevalence of anxiety and anxious depression—where symptoms of both anxiety and depression co-occur—have also been reported among lonely people (Heikkinen & Kauppinen, 2011). A recent cross-sectional Nigerian study confirmed these findings among older adults with 21.8% identified as lonely, 52% depressed, 27.7% anxious and 20.5% anxious depressed (Igbokwe et al., 2020).

Loneliness in later life has also been linked to cognitive decline, including dementia (Sutin et al., 2020). A recent Swedish longitudinal study examined the effect of self-reported loneliness on the development of all types of dementia, (Sundström et al., 2020). They found an increased risk of dementia of all types, specifically of Alzheimer's disease, except for vascular dementia. However, there is evidence that the effects of loneliness on cognition can be mitigated or reversed. For example, a Finnish study comparing social stimulation through group activities including art and creative writing, found improved cognition after 3 months and mental function at 12 months relative to a control group (Pitkala et al., 2011). Similar improvements in cognition relative to a control group have recently been reported from a music intervention that includes singing, songwriting, and socializing (Dingle et al., 2020: see also Chap. 7).

The importance of staying connected for human health and well-being cannot be overstated. Individuals such as Mrs Adeniyi who is living in Nigeria, far from family, hampered by mobility problems and limited financial resources, help us understand that as we age, multiple factors interact to interfere with staying connected. The different factors introduced in this chapter, including social isolation, staying connected to family friends and community, leisure activities and health, are explored further in subsequent chapters. But first, the next chapter introduces the types of AgeTech that are currently available and emerging to promote staying connected in later life. These are further explored in the subsequent chapters.

References

Andrews, J., Brown, L. J., Hawley, M., & Astell, A. J. (2019). Older adults' perspectives on using digital technology to maintain good mental health: Interactive group study. *Journal of Medical Internet Research, 21*(2), e11694.

Baez, M., Nielek, R., Casati, F., & Wierzbicki, A. (2019). Technologies for promoting social participation in later life. In B. Neves, & F. Vetere (Eds.) *Ageing and digital technology*. Springer.

Berg-Weger, M., & Morley, J. E. (2020). Loneliness in old age: An unaddressed health problem. *Journal of Nutrition, Health & Aging, 24*, 243–245. https://doi.org/10.1007/s12603-020-1323-6

Bornstein, M. H., Putnick, D. L., Rigo, P., et al. (2017). Culturally common maternal responses to infant cry. *Proceedings of the National Academy of Sciences, 114*(45), E9465–E9473. https://doi.org/10.1073/pnas.1712022114

Cacioppo, J. T., Hughes, M. E., Waite, L. J., Hawkley, L. C., et al. (2006). Loneliness as a specific risk factor for depressive symptoms: Cross-sectional and longitudinal analyses. *Psychology of Aging, 21*(1), 140–151.

Campaign to End Loneliness. (2015). Risk factors. Fact Sheet. Available at: https://campaigntoendloneliness.org/guidance/wp-content/uploads/2015/06/Risk-factorsGFLA.pdf

Dingle, G. A., Ellem, R. J., Davidson, R., et al. (2020). Pilot randomized controlled trial of the Live Wires music program for older adults living in a retirement village. *Journal of Music, Health and Well-Being* 1–19.

Hanratty, B., Stow, D., Collingridge Moore, D., et al. (2018). Loneliness as a risk factor for care home admission in the English longitudinal study of ageing. *Age and Ageing, 47*(6), 896–900. https://doi.org/10.1093/ageing/afy095

Heikkinen, R. L., & Kauppinen, M. (2011). Mental well-being: A 16-year follow-up among older residents in Jyvaskyla. *Archives of Gerontology & Geriatrics, 52*(1), 33–39.

Igbokwe, C. C., Ejeh, V. J., Agbaje, O. S. et al. (2020). Prevalence of loneliness and association with depressive and anxiety symptoms among retirees in Northcentral Nigeria: A cross-sectional study. *BMC Geriatrics, 20*(153). https://doi.org/10.1186/s12877-020-01561-4

Lee, S. L., Pearce, E., Ajnakina, O., et al. (2021). The association between loneliness and depressive symptoms among adults aged 50 years and older: A 12-year population-based cohort study. *Lancet: Psychiatry, 8*(1), 48–57.

Lowenthal, M. F. (1964). Social isolation and mental illness in old age. *American Sociological Review, 29*(1), 54–70.

Luo, Y., Hawkley, L. C., Waite, L. J., & Cacioppo, J. T. (2012). Loneliness, health, and mortality in old age: A national longitudinal study. *Social Science and Medicine, 74*(6), 907–914. https://doi.org/10.1016/j.socscimed.2011.11.028

Mann, R., Rabiee, P., Birks, Y., & Wilberforce, M. (2020). Identifying loneliness and social isolation in care home residents with sight loss: Lessons from using the De Jong Gierveld Scale. *Journal of Long-Term Care* 167–173.

Murthy, V. (2017). Work and the loneliness epidemic. Harvard Business Review, September 2017. Retrieved from: https://www.vivekmurthy.com/single-post/2017/10/10/Work-and-the-Loneliness-Epidemic-Harvard-Business-Review

Musich, S., Wang, S. S., Hawkins, K., & Yeh, C. S. (2015). The impact of loneliness on quality of life and patient satisfaction among older, sicker adults. *Gerontology and Geriatric Medicine*. https://doi.org/10.1177/2333721415582119

Neves, B. B., Sanders, A., & Kokanović, R. (2019). "It's the worst bloody feeling in the world": Experiences of loneliness and social isolation among older people living in care homes. *Journal of Aging Studies, 49*, 74–84. https://doi.org/10.1016/j.jaging.2019.100785

Nicholson, N. (2009). Social isolation in older adults: An evolutionary concept analysis. *Journal of Advanced Nursing, 65*, 1342–1352.

Paul, E., Bu, F., & Fancourt, D. (2021). Loneliness and risk for cardiovascular disease: mechanisms and future directions. *Current Cardiology Reports, 23*(6), 1–7. https://doi.org/10.1007/s11886-021-01495-2. PMID: 33961131; PMCID: PMC8105233.

Perissinotto, C. M., Cenzer, I. S., & Covinsky, K. E. (2012). Loneliness in older persons: A predictor of functional decline and death. *Archives of Internal Medicine, 172*(14), 1078–1084.

Perlman, D., & Peplau, L. A. (1981). Toward a social psychology of loneliness. *Personal Relationships, 3*, 31–56.

Pitkala, K. H., Routasalo, P., Kautiainen, H., et al. (2011). Effects of socially stimulating group intervention on lonely, older people's cognition: A randomized, controlled trial. *American Journal of Geriatric Psychiatry, 19*(7), 654–663.

Ruggles, S. (2001). Living arrangements and well-being of older persons in the past. *Population Bulletin of the United Nations, 42*, 111–161.

Ruggles, S. (2007). The decline of intergenerational co-residence in the United States, 1850 to 2000. *American Sociological Review, 72*(6), 964–989.

Ryan, R. M., & Deci, E. L. (2000). Self-Determination theory and the facilitation of intrinsic motivation, social development, and well-being. *American Psychologist, 55*(1), 68–78.

Savage, R. D, Wu, W., Li. J, et al. (2021). Loneliness among older adults in the community during COVID-19: A cross-sectional survey in Canada. *BMJ Open.* e044517. https://doi.org/10.1136/bmjopen-2020-044517

Sepúlveda-Loyola, W., Rodríguez-Sánchez, I., Pérez-Rodríguez, P., et al. (2020). Impact of social isolation due to COVID-19 on health in older people: Mental and physical effects and recommendations. *The Journal of Nutrition, Health & Aging*, 1–10. https://doi.org/10.1007/s12603-020-1469-2

Shukla, A., Harper, M., Pedersen, E., Goman, A., et al. (2020). Hearing loss, loneliness, and social isolation: A systematic review. *Otolaryngology–Head and Neck Surgery, 162*(5), 622–633. https://doi.org/10.1177/0194599820910377

Sundström, A., Nordin Adolfsson, A., Nordin, M., & Adolfsson, R. (2020). Loneliness increases the risk of all-cause dementia and Alzheimer's Disease. *The Journals of Gerontology: Series B, 75*(5), 919–926. https://doi.org/10.1093/geronb/gbz139

Sutin, A. R., Stephan, Y., Luchetti, M., & Terracciano, A. (2020). Loneliness and risk of dementia. *The Journals of Gerontology: Series B, 75*(7), 1414–1422.

United Nations, Department of Economic and Social Affairs, Population Division. (2017). Living arrangements of older persons: A report on an expanded international dataset (ST/ESA/SER.A/407). Available at: https://www.un.org/en/development/desa/population/publications/pdf/ageing/LivingArrangements.pdf

Vansteenkiste, M., Ryan, R. M., & Soenens, B. (2020). Basic psychological need theory: Advancements, critical themes and future directions. *Motivation and Emotion, 44*(1), 1–31.

Victor, C. R. (2012). Loneliness in care homes: A neglected area of research? *Aging and Health, 8*(6), 637–646. https://doi.org/10.2217/ahe.12.65

Ward, M., May, P., Normand, C., Kenny, R. A., & Nolan, A. (2021). Mortality risk associated with combinations of loneliness and social isolation. Findings from The Irish Longitudinal Study on Ageing (TILDA). *Age and Ageing*, 1329–1335. https://doi.org/10.1093/ageing/afab004

Wu, B. (2020). Social isolation and loneliness among older adults in the context of COVID-19: A global challenge. *Global Health Research & Policy, 5*(27), 1–3. https://doi.org/10.1186/s41256-020-00154-3

AgeTech for Staying Connected 3

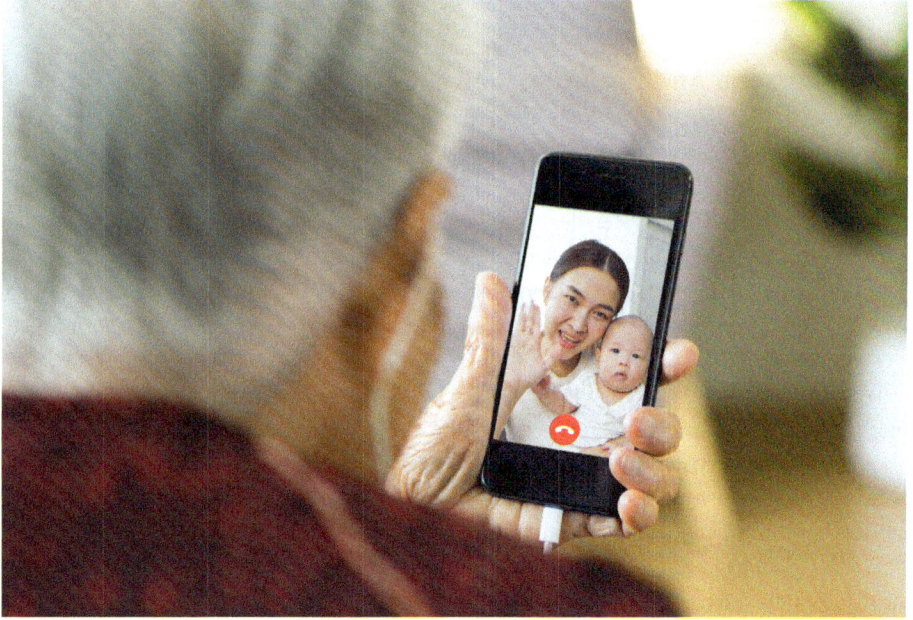

Image 3.1 *Credit* Shutterstock—Nattakorn Maneerat

3.1 The Challenge

Technology has long played a role in enabling people to stay connected. Before Alexander Graham Bell invented the telephone in 1876, the telegraph had been providing a way to send messages from one person to another since the 1830s (Telecommunications History Group, 2018). Today the potential for technology-mediated connections is greater than at any time, with multiple channels (e.g., voice, text, emojis, photographs, and video-calls) and devices (e.g., phones, computers, robots, virtual reality, and augmented reality) (Image 3.1). While many mainstream applications and devices are suitable for anyone to use, the number of applications, services and devices targeting the needs of older adults is growing. In this chapter, we briefly introduce the main AgeTech areas that will be considered in greater detail in subsequent chapters. First, we introduce Wen, an older lady living alone in Shanghai, China, managing multiple health conditions and feeling disconnected from her family and community.

3.2 Persona and Scenario: Wen[1]

Persona: Wen is a 92-year-old woman who lives alone in Shanghai. She has low blood pressure, rheumatoid arthritis and visual impairment, frequent dizziness and tinnitus, and pain in her back and arms. Her husband died a year ago and she misses him very much. She had three sons, her oldest son died a few years ago, her second-born son is a company leader, and her youngest son is a community worker. Although she now lives alone, she lives in the same neighbourhood as her youngest son, who visits her every morning and every evening.

Wen, with a pension of more than 4000 yuan (US$619) each month, has applied for long-term care insurance. The nursing assistant visits Wen twice a week, and she receives a bottle of milk every day from the state plus food delivery services from the community.

Sometimes Wen feels lonely because no one talks to her. She plans to move into a nursing home in the future. "My husband and I were married for more than 60 years," Wen said. "We have never scolded each other, but he's passed away, and I'm all alone and I feel lonely. My children want to find a care worker to take care of me but I don't want to. I usually turn on the TV and make a little noise in my house, as if someone is with me."

Wen didn't tell her children that she often got injured at home because she didn't want to make them worried. For example, once she slipped while taking a bath, and another time she knocked over the radio from a high place and hurt her head. There are always some bruises on her body without knowing where they are from. Fortunately, the accidents haven't done her much harm, but the risk of living alone is getting too high. Wen said that

---

[1] Case study created by Dr Fang Yang, Associate Professor, Department of Social Work, School of Sociology and Political Science, Shanghai University.

she was used to living alone, but she felt living in such a large apartment was a waste. Currently, Wen still can take care of herself. She often goes shopping independently, and she is very friendly and always on the balcony to wave goodbye to her friends who come to visit her.

Wen believes that supporting older adults increases the burden on the country and supporting older adults at home also increases the burden on the children. However, supporting older adults at home means that the children make contributions to the country to share the national pension pressure.

Scenario: While Wen is a very typical older person in China, her situation will be familiar across the world. As a widow, she is living alone, having recently lost her husband of many years. Unsurprisingly many people who lose a long-term partner and companion, experience feelings of loneliness when they no longer have someone around to speak to. Adjusting to such a major life change takes time, and people may need assistance to process the impact this has on all aspects of their lives. Most obvious is the absence of another person in their home. While some people have longer to prepare for this, for example, if their partner moves into a long-term care setting, the change in a person's status and identity, from being a partner to a single person, is still a large adjustment to make. There are also changes to the daily routine and activities, as the bereaved person takes over tasks that their partner previously carried out. Among the oldest-old (i.e., aged 80 and over) loss of a spouse or child, leads to a greater decline in daily functioning and longer-lasting symptoms of depression (d'Epinay et al., 2019). For people who have access to support from family and friends, social participation can help mitigate the loss, but this is not available to everyone (Utz et al., 2002).

Wen's heart disease causes dizziness which puts her at risk of falls and other accidents. She does not want to share these difficulties with her family, perhaps like many older people because she does not want to be a burden to portray an image of dependency (Astell et al., 2020). Also like many older people, Wen uses the television (some people use the radio) to create some sound in her home. However, she does not use many other technologies, such as a computer, smartphone, or tablet, which reduces her access to many online services and resources. Connecting Wen to her family and healthcare as well as some activities or groups for older adults could help her to feel less lonely and increase her agency over the situation. In the rest of this chapter, we briefly consider some of the commonly used AgeTech and the potential for keeping older adults such as Wen connected.

3.3 Types of AgeTech for Staying Connected

3.3.1 Internet

Accessing the Internet is becoming a necessity in many parts of the world as more and more daily activities, such as banking and shopping, move online. Many services such as healthcare appointments and renewing prescriptions as well as contacting local authorities or applying for government benefits are being completed online. Accessing the Internet can reduce loneliness through social interactions with family and friends (Cotton et al., 2013). The Internet is essential for older adults to access a wide range of resources, services, leisure and recreation pursuits, and social interaction. Examples of web-based resources such as online gaming, cultural visits, social platforms, and healthcare tools will be examined in subsequent chapters.

3.3.2 Videoconferencing

The COVID-19 pandemic escalated the use of video-conferencing platforms, bringing video calls into millions of homes. Popular apps such as WhatsApp, Zoom, Skype and WeChat, provide instant video calling to connect older adults with family, friends, and community groups. Simple to use apps such as WhatsApp and WeChat, combine multiple functions including sharing photos, sending texts, and commenting with emojis, alongside audio and video calls all in one place. The ease of use and functionality make these apps highly accessible and popular among older adults (Fernández-Ardèvol & Rosales, 2018) (Image 3.2).

The familiarity of videoconferencing extends to other activities that can keep people connected to social and recreational activities. The COVID-19 pandemic saw the emergence of many creative uses of videoconferencing including attending concerts and theatre productions, interactive magic shows, murder mysteries and stand-up comedy. Exercise and yoga classes, dancing and singing have all become available via videoconferencing (see Chap. 7), with many organizations planning to offer hybrid models of live and online in future (Lilley, 2020). This opens up many opportunities for older adults to socialize and stay connected to multiple activities and people.

3.3.3 Conversational Agents

Conversational agents or chatbots are computer systems designed to interact with humans through speech but also text, graphics, haptics (touch), and gestures. The intention is to provide a dialogue using natural language that simulates a conversation with another human. Chatbots are becoming ubiquitous in many services as they provide immediate

3.3 Types of AgeTech for Staying Connected

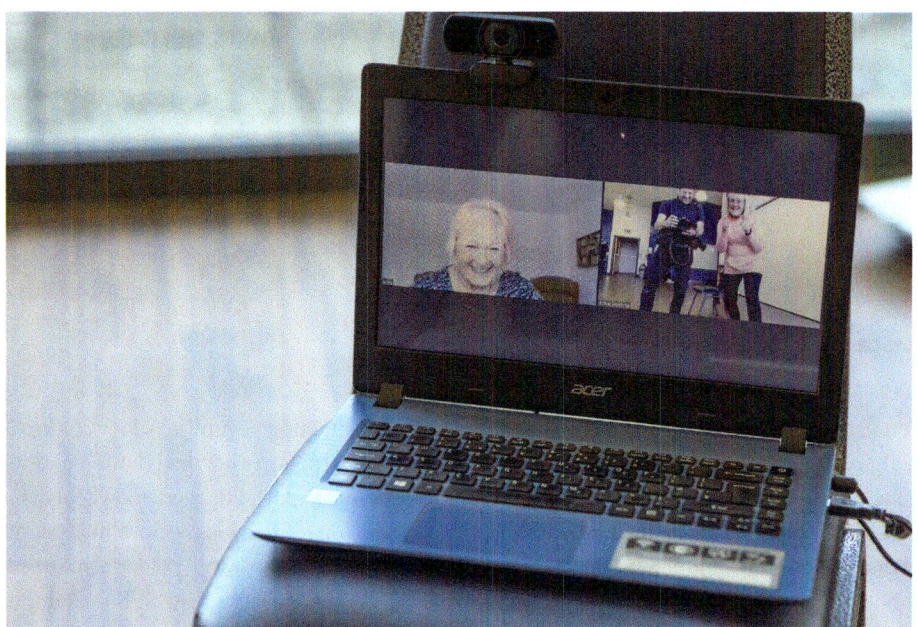

Image 3.2 *Credit* In-Press Photography/ageing better

responses to human inquiries and are available 24/7. One aspect of particular relevance to other adults is the growth of chatbots as a tool for staying connected to healthcare. In Chap. 9 we consider various healthcare chatbots and how they are supporting older adults to self-manage various common conditions of later life.

Voice-activated systems such as Amazon's Alexa, Apple's Siri and Google Home Hub have become increasingly popular for home-based Internet access. Voice control makes them particularly accessible for people with mobility restrictions and visual impairment as they can be used to control other devices in the home. Voice-activated systems are also very accessible for people with no prior computer experience. The range of applications and services that can be accessed via voice control offers useful functionality for older adults such as voice dialling, controlling environmental systems and functioning as 'smart assistants' (Ho, 2018). However, the potential of these systems for supporting active aging and staying connected is only starting to be explored (e.g. Astell & Clayton, 2024; Kowalski et al., 2019).

3.3.4 Robots

Whilst robots are commonly discussed in the context of making up gaps in the caregiving workforce for older people, their actual use has been most investigated in terms of staying

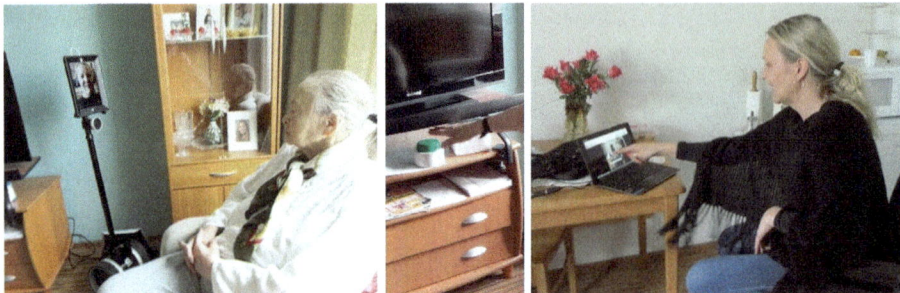

Image 3.3 *Credit* Niemelä et al. (2019)

connected. While care robots are usually the focus of attention regarding older adults, in reality, telepresence robots are the type that have been most investigated for potential benefits. Telepresence robots are essentially screens on a pole attached to wheels that can be remote-controlled to move around. Developed for business use—to allow people attending meetings remotely to have a 'presence' in the room—the potential of these robots for supporting older adults has been investigated in a variety of ways. For example, research has looked at telepresence robots delivering remote visits to older adults' homes for healthcare, such as monitoring wound care of an older adult in a remote location (Vaughn et al., 2015) and social interaction, e.g., connecting with family (Image 3.3; Niemelä et al., 2019).

In this study, the care home resident had the telepresence robot in their room (left image). There was a separate (green) button to request a family member to connect via SMS (middle image). The family member connected using a laptop (right image) (Niemelä et al., 2019).

3.3.5 Virtual Reality

Virtual Reality (VR) is an environment containing scenes and objects generated by a computer to create an immersive experience for the user. VR environments are perceived through a headset which permits the user to 'engage' in a wide range of activities. In VR environments users can interact with objects and people, making it popular as a game platform. However, the potential to simulate actual interactions has also led to VR being explored for a wide range of learning scenarios from heart surgery (see Sadeghi et al., 2020)[2] to training by both the US Army[3] and Navy.[4]

---

[2] https://www.youtube.com/watch?v=x9D9eIWZNgM
[3] https://www.youtube.com/watch?v=E6SfnRhEiTQ
[4] https://www.youtube.com/watch?v=JIgeMJx4g0c

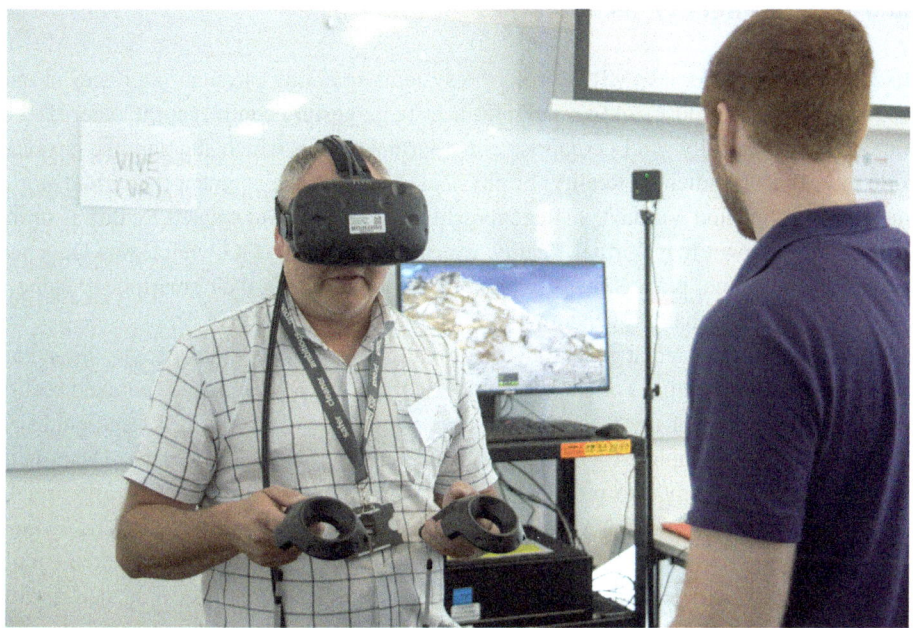

Image 3.4 *Credit* Simon Butler/University of Sheffield

VR has also been used for the treatment of mental health conditions including anxiety (Maples-Keller et al., 2017), schizophrenia (Bisso et al., 2020) and post-traumatic stress disorder (PTSD) (Kothgassner et al., 2019). In the UK, the NHS has been trialling VR treatments for social anxiety, pain reduction during burn treatments and to relax patients during minor surgery. Applications of VR targeting later life include 'A walk through dementia', an educational film developed by Alzheimer's Research UK, to provide insights into what it is like to live with dementia.[5] Similarly, EDIE Educational Dementia Immersive Experience is a training program developed by Dementia Australia based on the experience of living with dementia[6] (Image 3.4).

VR has also been used as an intervention to reduce older adult's risk of falling (Cho et al., 2014) and improve balance (de Amorim et al., 2018). Condition-specific applications include stroke and Parkinson's Disease, although recent reviews suggest that the evidence in both populations is not as strong or clear as it needs to be for widespread recommendation: (For stroke Cochrane review see Laver et al., 2017 and PD review see Canning et al., 2020).

---

[5] https://www.youtube.com/watch?v=R-Rcbj_qR4g

[6] https://www.dementia.org.au/information/resources/technology/edie

3.3.6 Mixed Reality Technologies

Mixed reality technologies (MRTs) describe systems spanning physical interfaces at one end (e.g., computer mouse) and virtual interfaces (e.g., gesture control) at the other (Desai et al., 2016). Essentially MRTs comprise either virtual objects which augment the physical world (so-called Augmented Reality) or physical objects which augment the virtual world (known as Augmented Virtuality) (Regenbrecht et al., 2004). Augmented Reality is probably less well-known than Virtual Reality, except for Pokémon GO, which was launched in 2016. In this game, players travel around their vicinity using their smartphone camera to 'catch' Pokémons that are generated by the GPS of the location.

AR technology has great potential for providing support to older people, including those living with dementia. For example, the HoloLens from Microsoft is a mixed reality device that is capable of tracking people's gaze whilst they carry out tasks and could be used to detect when people go off track during an activity (Desai et al., 2020). The system could also be programmed to provide prompts to get them back on track at appropriate times. Similarly, Augmented Virtuality technologies, such as Kinect and Osmo, which are primarily used for leisure and recreation (see Chap. 7), could also track people's behaviour, and provide feedback during games or other activities. As indicated above, there exist multiple challenges for accessing and leveraging all of the potential benefits of AgeTech for staying connected some of which will be discussed in Chap. 10.

3.4 Key Initiative #VoiceforLoneliness

#VoiceforLoneliness was set up to examine the potential of voice-activated technology for older adults living alone. Established as a collaboration between Abbeyfield, a UK housing and care provider and Greenwood Campbell, a UK technology company, #VoiceForLoneliness provided smart speakers to older adults living in residential accommodation for eight weeks. Collaborating with researchers from the University of Reading, the study examined the impact of smart speakers on older adults' sense of isolation and loneliness. This study demonstrated the feasibility and benefits of older adults utilizing smart speakers to alleviate feelings of loneliness and lack of company (Astell & Clayton, 2024).

References

Astell, A. J., McGrath, C., & Dove, E. (2020). "That's for old so and so's!" Does identity influence older adults' technology adoption decisions? *Ageing and Society, 40*, 1550–1576.

Astell, A., & Clayton, D. (2024). "Like another human being in the room": A community case study of smart speakers to reduce loneliness in the oldest-old. *Frontier in Psychology, 15*, 1320555. https://doi.org/10.3389/fpsyg.2024.1320555

References

Bisso, E., Signorelli, M. S., Milazzo, M., et al. (2020). Immersive virtual reality applications in schizophrenia spectrum therapy: A systematic review. *International Journal of Environmental Research and Public Health, 17*(17), 6111. https://doi.org/10.3390/ijerph17176111

Canning, C. G., Allen, N. E., Nackaerts, E., et al. (2020). Virtual reality in research and rehabilitation of gait and balance in Parkinson's disease. *Nature Reviews Neurology, 16*, 409–425. https://doi.org/10.1038/s41582-020-0370-2

Cho, G. H., Hwangbo, G., & Shin, H. S. (2014). The effects of virtual reality-based balance training on balance of the elderly. *The Journal of Physical Therapy Science, 26*(4), 615–617.

Cotten, S. R., Anderson, W. A., & McCullough, B. M. (2013). Impact of internet use on loneliness and contact with others among older adults: Cross-sectional analysis. *Journal of Medical Internet Research, 15*(2), 1–13. https://doi.org/10.2196/jmir.2306

de Amorim, J. S. C., Leite, R. C., Brizola, R. et al. (2018). Virtual reality therapy for rehabilitation of balance in the elderly: A systematic review and META-analysis. *Advances in Rheumatology, 58*, (18). https://doi.org/10.1186/s42358-018-0013-0

d'Epinay, C. J., Cavalli, S., Guillet, L. A. (2019). Bereavement in very old age: Impact on health and relationships of the loss of a spouse, a child, a sibling, or a close friend. *Omega (Westport), 60*(4), 301–25. https://doi.org/10.2190/om.60.4.a. PMID: 20397613

Desai, S., Blackler, A., Fels, D., & Astell, A. (2020). Supporting people with dementia: Understanding their interactions with Mixed Reality Technologies. *Proceedings of Design Research Society International Conference, 2020*, 615–637.

Desai, S., Blackler, A., & Popovic, V. (2016). Intuitive interaction in a mixed reality system. In P. Lloyd, & E. Bohemia, (Eds.), *Future focused thinking—DRS international conference 2016*, 27–30 June, Brighton, United Kingdom. https://doi.org/10.21606/drs.2016.369

Fernández-Ardèvol, M., & Rosales, A. (2018). Older people, smartphones and WhatsApp. In J. Vincent, & Haddon, L. (Eds.), *Smartphone cultures*. Routledge

Ho, D. K. (2018). Voice-controlled virtual assistants for the older people with visual impairment. *Eye, 32*(1), 53–54. https://doi.org/10.1038/eye.2017.165

Kothgassner, O. D., Goreis, A., Kafka, J. X., Van Eickels, R. L., et al. (2019). Virtual reality exposure therapy for posttraumatic stress disorder (PTSD): A meta-analysis. *European Journal of Psychotraumatology, 10*(1), 1654782. https://doi.org/10.1080/20008198.2019.1654782

Kowalski, J., Skorupska, K., Kopeć, W., Jakulska, A., et al. (2019). Older adults and voice interaction: A pilot study with Google Home. *ArXiv.1903.07195*. https://arxiv.org/pdf/1903.07195.pdf

Laver, K. E., Lange, B., George, S., Deutsch J.E., et al. (2017). Virtual reality for stroke rehabilitation. *Cochrane Database of Systematic Reviews*, 11. Art. No.: CD008349. https://doi.org/10.1002/14651858.CD008349.pub4

Lilley, M. (2020). Has 2020 given us a new hybrid model of performance? https://www.theatreartlife.com/artistic/has-2020-given-us-a-new-hybrid-model-of-performance/

Maples-Keller, J. L., Bunnell, B. E., Kim, S. J., & Rothbaum, B. O. (2017). The use of virtual reality technology in the treatment of anxiety and other psychiatric disorders. *Harvard Review of Psychiatry, 25*(3), 103–113. https://doi.org/10.1097/HRP.0000000000000138

Niemelä, M., van Aerschot, L., Tammela, A., Aaltonen, I., et al. (2019). Towards ethical guidelines of using telepresence robots in residential care. *International Journal of Social Robotics*, 1–9. https://doi.org/10.1007/s12369-019-00529-8

Regenbrecht, H., Lum, T., Kohler, P., Ott, C., et al. (2004). Using augmented virtuality for remote collaboration. *Presence: Teleoperators and Virtual Environments, 13*(3), 338–354. https://doi.org/10.1162/1054746041422334

Sadeghi, A. H., Bakhuis, W., Van Schaagen, F., Oei, F. B. S., et al. (2020). Immersive 3D virtual reality imaging in planning minimally invasive and complex adult cardiac surgery. *European Heart Journal Digital Health, 1*(1), 62–70. https://doi.org/10.1093/ehjdh/ztaa011

Telecommunications History Group 1800–1900. (2018). Available at http://www.telcomhistory.org/?s=telegraph

Utz, R. L., Carr, D., Nesse, R., & Wortman, C. B. (2002). The effect of widowhood on older adults' social participation: An evaluation of activity, disengagement, and continuity theories. *The Gerontologist, 42*(4), 522–533. https://doi.org/10.1093/geront/42.4.522

Vaughn, J., Shaw, R. J., & Molloy, M. A., (2015). A telehealth case study. *Journal of the American Psychiatric Nurses Association, 21*, 431–432. https://doi.org/10.1177/1078390315617037

Supporting Social Interaction with Existing Social Networks 4

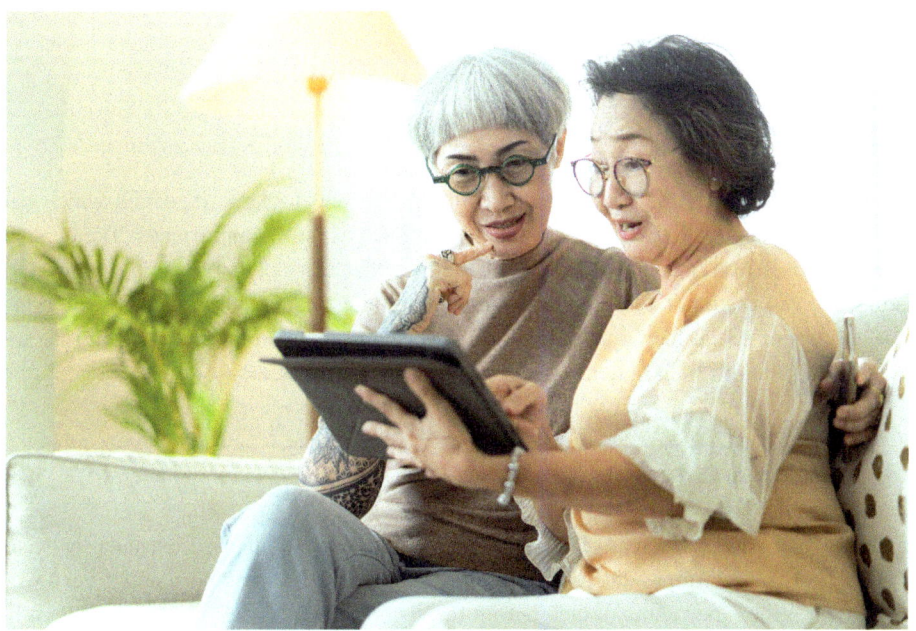

Image 4.1 *Credit* Shutterstock—WHYFRAME

4.1 The Challenge

As described in Chap. 2, being connected to other people is a fundamental component of being human. Our sense of self—that is our experience of being a person in the world—is provided by and reinforced through our interactions with others from the moment we are born. Other people responding and reacting to us, recognizing us as fellow humans in the social world, are important contributors to mental health and well-being (Image 4.1). In early life, we are surrounded by people to interact with, and this continues into adulthood. As we progress from school to work or university, our opportunities to meet new people and grow our social networks increase. For a period of time, family may become the major source of social interaction, until children grow up and set out on their own. In later life, while there is more time to participate in activities outside the home, health, economic resources, location, or living situation may all contribute to reduced opportunities for social interaction. However, engaging in social interaction either in person or remotely through phone, messaging or video-calling is essential for well-being.

4.2 What's in This Chapter?

This chapter addresses the need for social interaction and looks at AgeTech which can facilitate connection with existing social networks such as family and friends. The persona and scenario of Maria demonstrate the challenges that can occur in staying connected, leading to a discussion of a range of modern technologies that can offer creative solutions. Also, the use of social media and online social networks, including digital platforms and activities to promote social interaction directed at older adults.

4.3 Persona and Scenario: Maria

Persona: Maria is an 84-year-old lady living in a nursing home in Ensenada, Mexico. After her husband Enrique died, her children noticed that she was not coping very well on her own. When they came to pick her up for visits to their homes, they noticed that the house was becoming untidy and that housework was left undone. Maria, who had always paid attention to her appearance when going out, was often wearing clothes that needed washing and had not brushed her hair. The family also became concerned that Maria was not eating regularly and seemed to be confused about the time of day. This led them to consult their doctor and following an assessment, Maria was diagnosed with Alzheimer's disease. The doctor suggested this was not a recent problem and that Enrique had probably taken over household tasks before he died, as Maria became unable to do them. His death revealed the extent of her difficulties to her family, who had not been aware Maria was having problems. To provide the support she needed, Maria's two daughters and her son and daughter-in-law developed a rota to visit her several times a day, where they would bring food and help her with household chores. Over time, Maria's needs for care and support increased and the family realised that she needed to have full-time care. None of her family was in a position to have Maria move in with them, so they sought out a nursing home that could provide the care she needed.

Scenario: Maria moved into a government run care home where she shares a room with another lady also living with dementia. As in many parts of the world, the staffing levels in the nursing home mean that there is little one-to-one time with residents. At first, Maria wants to go home and often walks around the nursing home looking for Enrique. She tells the staff that she has to go home to make dinner for her children when they come in from school and becomes upset when they tell her that she has to stay in the nursing home. When this happens, they take her to her room and if she is particularly distressed, they administer antipsychotic medication to calm her down. As time passes, Maria becomes withdrawn and her family are concerned that she is lonely in the nursing home, even though there are many people around.

Solution: Professor Jesus Favela and Dr Dogoberto Cruz-Sandoval work in the Computer Science department at The Center for Scientific Research and Higher Education at Ensenada (Cruz-Sandoval et al. 2020). They are creating a social robot called Eva to help staff in nursing homes use alternatives to drugs in their care of people like Maria who are living with dementia. Eva is a tabletop robot designed to carry out simple interactions automatically. For more complex interactions a human operator can remotely control Eva to send personal greetings to a resident and deliver different predefined verbal responses such as telling jokes. The remote controller can also get Eva to make different facial expressions of emotion. Finally, Eva can be controlled to search for and play music that the resident likes.

Cruz-Sandoval & Favela bring Eva to the nursing home and Maria's family are keen for her to be included in the research, which could make her less isolated. The robot Eva is brought to Maria's room and says "Hello, Maria". This gets Maria's attention, and she says "hello" back. Through the remote control, Eva then asks Maria what music she likes, and Maria says 'Cerezo Rosa' a popular song from the 1950s. Eva finds a version of Cerezo Rosa and plays it for Maria who smiles when the music starts and sings along. The next day the researchers return, and the staff invite Maria to come to the sitting room where Eva is set up for a small group session. Along with two other residents, Maria enjoys conversation and a singalong with Eva and a member of staff. Maria attends more sessions with Eva which she enjoys very much, chatting with the other residents, singing old songs, and reminiscing about their younger days (Image 4.2).

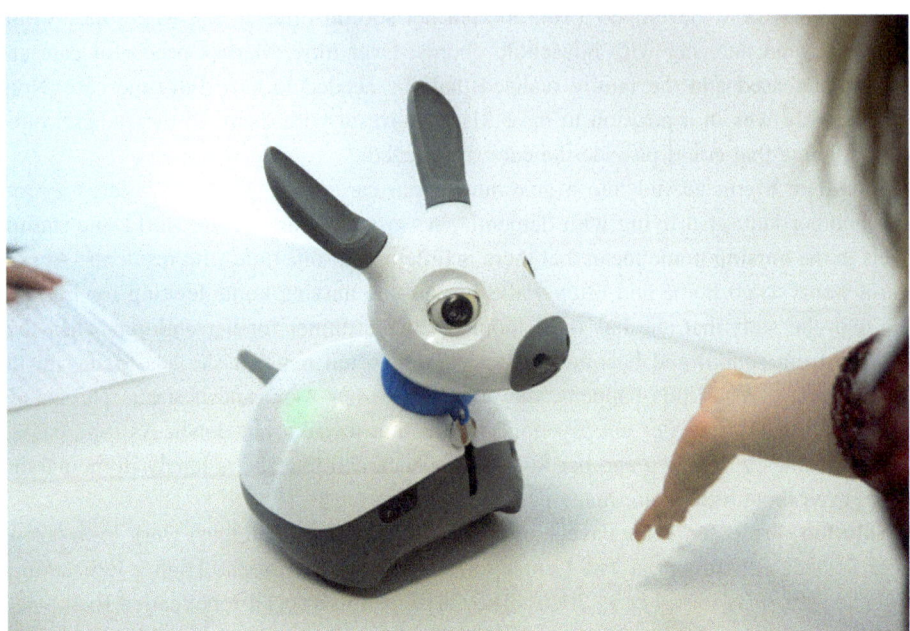

Image 4.2 Miro Robot.[1] *Credit* Simon Butler/University of Sheffield

4.4 Technology Solutions

4.4.1 Remote and Virtual Connections

Maria's case demonstrates how susceptible people living in care services can be to becoming disconnected. A review of studies that assessed loneliness in care home residents reported that the prevalence was at least double that of people living in the community (Victor, 2012). Consequently, many emerging technological solutions are focusing on the challenge of social isolation and loneliness for those living in long-term care services. For example, Baker et al. (2020) used the Oculus Rift system to deliver a range of creative and explorative virtual reality activities at a large long-term care facility in Melbourne, Australia. They aimed to engage residents for whom social isolation was caused by boredom with the usual facilitated activities and a perceived lack of commonality with their peers. Using qualitative research methods, they found evidence in support of the role that interactive virtual reality can have in engaging isolated residents. Sherish^{SM} Connect allows family and friends to create a shared photo album which can be easily viewed by an older person on their television. A small-scale evaluation of Sherish^{SM} by researchers at Huntington University in the USA reported promising results in terms of increasing social

---

[1] https://consequentialrobotics.com/miro-beta.

4.4 Technology Solutions

participation and reducing loneliness and social isolation for residents in care services (Bennett et al., 2021).

Promoting social interaction and engagement is also important for reducing the risk of depression and other mental and physical health problems. Devices such as Komp and a simple device created by AGE-WELL researchers at the Technologies for Aging Gracefully Lab (TAGlab) in Toronto are tackling this problem. TAGlab co-created an accessible tablet-based communication app with older adults at risk of social isolation and loneliness. Partnering with frail, older adults living in institutions who had no previous computer experience or other challenges, such as motor problems, that interfered with using devices (Neves et al., 2018). The app supports video, audio and image sharing and includes a 'wave' icon to let someone know a family member is thinking of them. The accessible interface is based on icons rather than text. From the feasibility study, Neve et al. found that 'older participants preferred to receive text and send audio messages probably due to their familiarity with the telephone and the written form' (p. 1694) (Image 4.3).

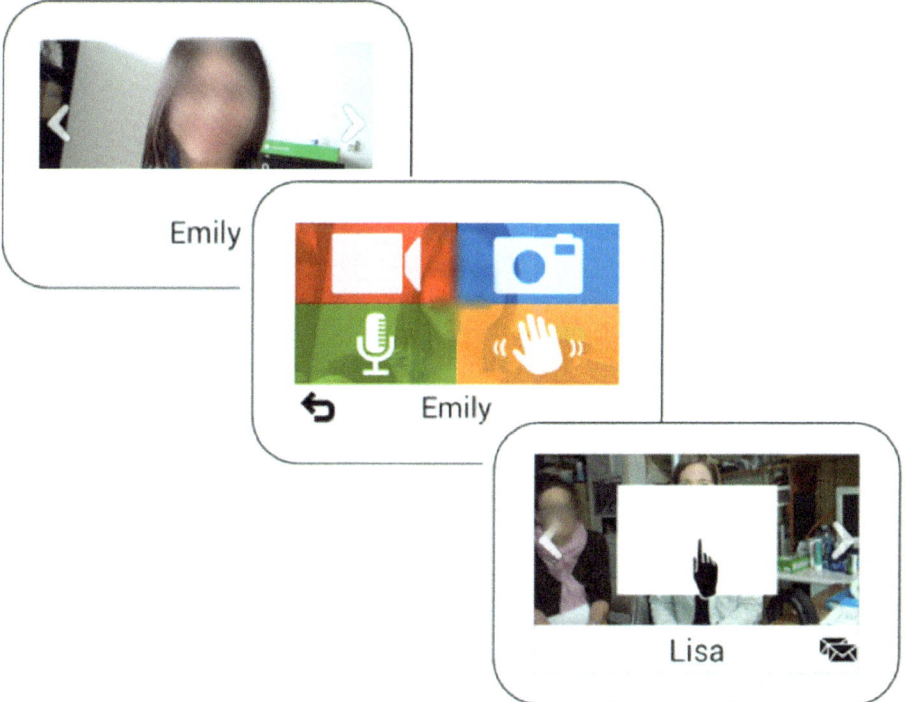

Image 4.3 *Credit* Barbosa Neves, B., and Baecker, R. (2022)

4.4.1.1 Telepresence Robots

As presented in the case of Maria, robots can be used to provide social support, but they can also be used in other contexts to address social isolation, such as facilitating remote connections through video calls in either private residences or care services. These mobile telepresence robots are designed to enhance the video-call service by enabling the caller to move around a remote location. Research by Niemelä et al. (2019) in Finland (introduced in Chap. 3) found that telepresence robots increased the sense of 'presence', and possibly also the engagement of family members in residential care. However, they identified privacy as a major concern due to the mobility of the telepresence robot. To address these concerns, the researchers proposed a set of ethical guidelines for the use of telepresence robots in long-term care services (to view the full guidelines, see the link in Sect. 4.6). These guidelines attempt to assign levels of acceptance to various applications of telepresence robots in residential care settings, the outcome of which can be summarised by the distinction between calls in private spaces of residents, which were well accepted, and calls in communal spaces, which were less well accepted. Privacy is less of a concern where users are living in their own homes, or at least the issues shift from the collective to the individual (Reinhardt et al., 2021), although the question of cost-effectiveness is raised when an individual is making a personal purchase (Isabet et al., 2021).

4.4.2 Social Media

Using existing online social networks to stay connected has also been explored. It is estimated that on average 1.62 billion users visit Facebook every day. Sinclair and Grieves (2017) examined the social connectedness of 280 Facebook users (25% male) aged between 55 and 81 predominantly from Australia, the United Kingdom, and Europe. They used the revised Facebook connectedness scale (Grieve et al., 2013) to measure how socially connected people feel on Facebook. They found that the…

> …older adults in this sample gained feelings of Facebook-derived connection similar to levels reported in younger samples in previous research' (Sinclair & Grieves, 2017, p. 367).

4.4.3 Digital Storytelling

Another tool for connecting is storytelling, which is a universal activity that serves many different functions. At its most basic, storytelling is a way of making connections and staying connected with other people (Fels & Astell, 2011). Benefits for older adults include staying connected through sharing experiences reminiscing and reflecting on their lives and creating a legacy (Hausknecht et al., 2019). AGE-WELL has supported several storytelling initiatives that are summarised here, including the move to an online platform of an established 10-week digital storytelling course for older adults (Schell et al., 2019). Another approach to using storytelling to connect families is Frame of Mind. This is an application that uses speech captured during storytelling to automatically organize photographs into "album-like" sets, to support family socialising (Axtell & Munteanu, 2018).

Digital storytelling has also been explored as a vehicle for connecting older adults with younger generations in Indigenous communities. AGE-WELL funded a pilot project to design and evaluate an intergenerational digital storytelling workshop to bring together Elders and school children from a First Nations community in Canada. In many First Nations communities, storytelling is a valued aspect of teaching and learning history, language, place, culture, and sharing indigenous knowledge. Over a 10-session program, 13 Elders were paired with 31 grade six and seven students with whom they shared stories, including personal experiences, legends, and local knowledge of hunting and medicine. The students created digital versions of the stories, from which they learnt local knowledge, built connections with Elders, and increased their digital literacy (Hausknecht et al., 2021).

Funding from AGE-WELL and the Canadian Consortium on Neurodegeneration and Aging, enabled digital storytelling to be extended to individuals living with dementia (Daum et al., 2019). Twenty-one individuals living with dementia in Alberta, British Columbia, and Ontario co-created digital stories with members of the research team. The research confirmed that people living with dementia can play an active role in co-creating stories of importance to them. The digital stories were shared with families, with a day program organising a cinema-style 'premiere' screening with popcorn and soft drinks. Sharing digital stories with families supports the social connections of people with dementia, as well as providing an important legacy (Liu et al., 2018). Storytelling is also incorporated into the collaborative Building Better Visits initiative, a collaboration between Dementia Australia, Lifeview Residential Care, and Swinburne University's Future Self and Design Living Lab. In Building Better Visits, Sonja Pedell and her colleagues used a tablet to improve communication between people living with dementia in long-term care and their visitors and found that the *'technology is providing cues to instigate rich storytelling and other conversations between the older adult and their visitors.'*

4.5 Key Initiative—Teledining

Eating together or 'commensality', is a fundamental of human social behavior (Fischler, 2011). Across cultures, mealtimes are essential for children to learn the ritual, social and emotional meanings of food and eating (Ochs & Shohat, 2006) In later life, eating together rather than alone has been shown to improve calorie intake (Wright et al., 2006)

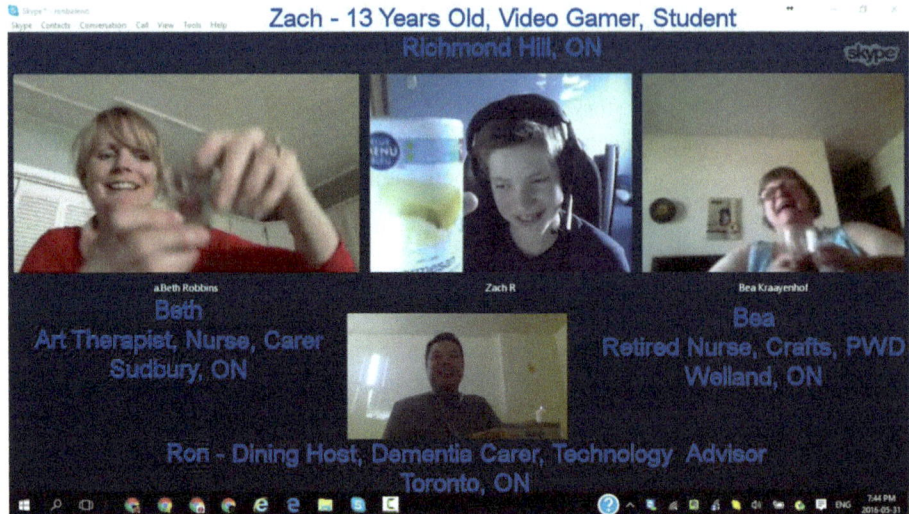

Image 4.4 *Credit* Ron Beleno

in addition to the social benefits. Videoconferencing technology has made dining with others very doable, but before the pandemic, there was little exploration of this as a means to help people stay connected. One early example is an initiative set up in Ontario, Canada bringing people living with dementia, caregivers, professionals, and volunteers to eat together on video (Image 4.4).

In 2014 Ron Beleno, a caregiver for his father living with Alzheimer's disease since 2007, attended the first Toronto Dementia Hackathon, an event funded by the UK Department of Trade and Industry to stimulate new products for people living with dementia. Also at the Dementia Hackathon was Bea Kraayenhof, a retired nurse living with dementia. Bea was a speaker at the event, discussing how she currently used technology and what she would like in future. At the subsequent 2015 Dementia Hackathon Ron and Bea reconnected and Ron was interested in whether Bea had received any new technology from the previous event. Finding that she hadn't, Ron set to thinking about what might benefit Bea.

Whilst caring for his father Ron had used Skype with auto-answering to see and speak to his dad remotely. Bea was already a confident tablet user, so Ron suggested they use Skype to connect as it was difficult for them to meet in person due to the distance they lived apart. Over time they started to eat 'together' in their own homes and were soon inviting one or two other people to join them. This included young people and professionals who were interested to meet Bea and share a meal. This was long before the pandemic brought social connecting into focus and as Ron says: 'There was no word for it, not teledining. We were just having meals together online. It was about connecting together.' (Interview with Ron Beleno, 25th June 2021).

4.6 Find Out More

- A useful summary about the importance of staying connected and tips for doing so provided by Independent Age in the UK: https://www.independentage.org/get-advice/wellbeing/relationships/staying-connected.
- Draft ethical guidelines for using a mobile telepresence robot in residential care for communication between residents and family members (Niemelä et al., 2019). https://link.springer.com/article/10.1007/s12369-019-00,529-8/tables/4.

References

Axtell, B., & Munteanu, C. (2018). Frame of mind: Using storytelling for speech-based clustering of family pictures. *IUI '18 Companion: Proceedings of the 23rd International Conference on Intelligent User Interfaces Companion, 22*, 1–2. https://doi.org/10.1145/3180308.3180330

Baker, S., Waycott, J., Robertson, E., Carrasco, R., Neves, B. B., et al. (2020). Evaluating the use of interactive virtual reality technology with older adults living in residential aged care. *Information Processing and Management, 57*(3), 1–13. https://doi.org/10.1016/j.ipm.2019.102105

Bennett, K., Gonzalez, M. L., Harper, S. L., Logan, M. N., et al. (2021). Effects of social technology on older adults in a residential living facility. *Student Journal of Occupational Therapy, 2*(2), 1–14. https://doi.org/10.46409/001.MCFL9362

Cruz-Sandoval, D., Morales-Tellez, A., Sandoval, E. B., & Favela, J. (2020). A social robot as therapy facilitator in interventions to deal with dementia-related behavioral symptoms. In *Proceedings of the 2020 ACM/IEEE international conference on human-robot interaction*, pp. 161–169. Association for Computing Machinery. https://doi.org/10.1145/3319502.3374840

Daum, C., Liu, L., Hollinda, K., Kaufman, D., & Astell, A. J. (2019). Skills and strategies of facilitators who co-create digital stories with persons with dementia. *Innovation in Aging, 3*(1), 453.

Fels, D. I., & Astell, A. J. (2011). Storytelling as a model of conversation for people with dementia and caregivers. *American Journal of Alzheimer's Disease and Other Dementias, 26*(7), 535–541.

Fischler, C. (2011). Commensality, society and culture. *Social Science Information, 50*(3–4), 528–548.

Grieve, R., Indian, M., Witteveen, K., Tolan, G. A., & Marrington, J. (2013). Face-to-face or Facebook: Can social connectedness be derived online? *Computers in Human Behaviour, 29*(3), 604–609.

Hausknecht, S., Vanchu-Orosco, M., & Kaufman, D. (2019). Digitising the wisdom of our elders: Connectedness through digital storytelling. *Ageing Society, 39*, 2714–2734. https://doi.org/10.1017/S0144686X18000739

Hausknecht, S., Freeman, S., Martin, J., Nash, C., & Skinner, K. (2021). Sharing Indigenous Knowledge through intergenerational digitals Storytelling: Design of a workshop engaging Elders and youth, Educational Gerontology, https://doi.org/10.1080/03601277.2021.1927484

Isabet, B., Pino, M., Lewis, M., Benveniste, S., & Rigaud, A. S. (2021). Social telepresence robots: A narrative review of experiments involving older adults before and during the COVID-19 pandemic. *International Journal of Environmental Research and Public Health, 18*(7), 3597. https://doi.org/10.3390/ijerph18073597

Liu, L., Owens, E., Park, E., Astell, A., Beleno, R., et al. (2018). Persons with dementia use digital storytelling to enhance memory, connect socially and leave legacies. *Innovation in Aging, 2*(1), 317–318.

Neves, B. B., Franz, R. L., Munteanu, C., & Baecker, R. (2018) Adoption and feasibility of a communication app to enhance social connectedness amongst frail institutionalized oldest old: An embedded case study. *Information, Communication and Society, 21*(11), 1681–1699. https://doi.org/10.1080/1369118X.2017.1348534

Niemelä, M., van Aerschot, L., Tammela, A., Aaltonen, I., & Lammi, H. (2019). Towards ethical guidelines of using telepresence robots in residential care. *International Journal of Social Robotics, 13*(3), 431–439. https://doi.org/10.1007/s12369-019-00529-8

Ochs, E., & Shohat, M. (2006). The cultural structuring of mealtime socialization. *New Directions for Child and Adolescent Development, 111*, 35–49. https://doi.org/10.1002/cad.153

Reinhardt, D., Khurana, M., & Hernández Acosta, L. (2021). "I still need my privacy": Exploring the level of comfort and privacy preferences of German-speaking older adults in the case of mobile assistant robots. *Pervasive and Mobile Computing, 74*. https://doi.org/10.1016/j.pmcj.2021.101397

Schell, R., da Silva, D., & Kaufman, D. (2019). Enhancing an online digital storytelling course for older adults through the Implementation of andragogical principles. In *Proceedings of the 11th international conference on computer supported education (CSEDU 219)*, pp. 313–320. https://doi.org/10.5220/0007579603130320

Sinclair, T. J., & Grieve, R. (2017). Facebook as a source of social connectedness in older adults. *Computers I Human Behaviour, 66*(1), 363–369.

Victor, C. R. (2012). Loneliness in care homes: A neglected area of research? *Aging and Health, 8*(6), 637–646. https://doi.org/10.2217/ahe.12.65

Wright, L., Hickson, M., & Frost, G. (2006). Eating together is important: Using a dining room in an acute elderly medical ward increases energy intake. *Journal of Human Nutrition and Diet, 19*(1), 23–6.

Social Isolation and Mental Well-Being 5

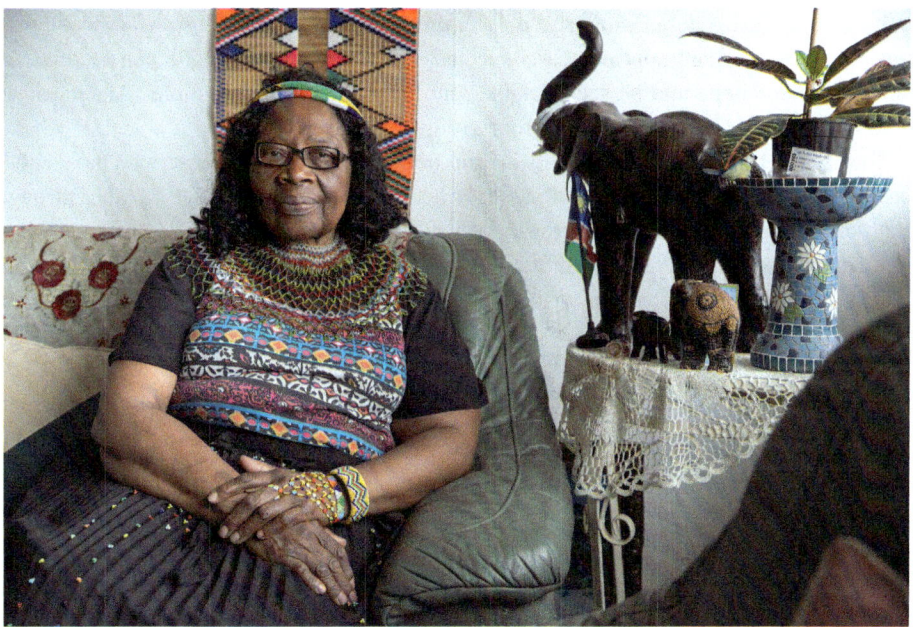

Image 5.1 *Credit* Independent Age/Leanne Benson

5.1 The Challenge

Our previous chapter on social interaction explored ways that technology can support people to find channels to connect with their existing social networks. In contrast, this chapter focuses on those people who for many different reasons might have become isolated from society, and who could use support to reconnect. Again, technology can play many different roles in this process; from being a conduit by which people can form new connections or relationships, all the way through to providing a presence within the home environment (Image 5.1).

The terms 'social isolation' and 'loneliness' are often confused, and sometimes even used interchangeably. However, there is a key difference that highlights the experiential nature of these concepts (Table 5.1).

Under these definitions, a person could be objectively considered to be socially isolated, yet if they were content with their situation, they may not wish to label themselves or be labelled, as lonely. Similarly, it is entirely possible that a person could be surrounded by people and appear well-connected socially from an outside perspective, yet feel completely alone and be seeking other, more meaningful connections. Andersson in 1998 captured these distinctions into four groups (Table 5.2).

Townsend (1957, 1973) made a distinction between 'desolates' (those who have either recently become disabled through illness or who had lost a close relative whether through death or migration) and 'isolates' (those with sustained little or no social contacts). Desolates were those isolated relative to their previous situations rather than because of having little contact with others in the past. His view was that older people who experienced loneliness were more likely to be 'desolates' rather than 'isolates'. Companionship for Townsend was important in older age. Loneliness was 'the unwelcome feeling of lack or loss of companionship' (Townsend, 1973, p. 256). This was most likely to be found where bereavement had deprived an older person of this companionship. This chapter is titled 'Social Isolation', as it offers people who are objectively isolated from society

Table 5.1 Definitions of isolation and loneliness

Social isolation	Loneliness
Objective state of having limited social contacts or interactions with other people	***Subjective*** experience of being alone, but with the desire to have interactions with other people

Table 5.2 Relationship between isolation and loneliness

	Isolated	Not isolated
Lonely	1. Being alone and feeling lonely	2. Not being alone but still feeling lonely
Not lonely	3. Being alone but not feeling lonely	4. Not being alone and not feeling lonely

After Andersson (1998)

opportunities to make connections with others, whether or not they consider themselves to be 'lonely'.

5.2 What's in This Chapter?

This chapter will demonstrate how technological innovation can be used to address the challenge of social isolation. The persona and scenario of Simon highlight how social isolation can emerge, with a focus on the relationship between staying connected and mental health. Several examples of digital services being used around the world to facilitate new connections between older adults and their community are presented, one of which is featured as this chapter's key initiative. The technologies and services featured in this chapter include chatbots, digital apps, and communication platforms.

5.3 Persona and Scenario: Simon

Persona: Simon is 67 years old and a retired carpenter and joiner living alone in a village in Northamptonshire in the UK. He and his wife Annie, a retired legal secretary, were enjoying an active retirement working in their garden: Simon successfully growing prize-winning dahlias and vegetables and Annie turning the fruit and vegetables into jams and pickles. Keen travellers, they were also enjoying rediscovering parts of the UK they had not visited since before they had a family. They had no children. However, ten months ago Annie was unexpectedly diagnosed with Stage 4 pancreatic cancer and died soon after. Annie was always more of an extrovert than Simon and arranged many of their social activities in the village. Since her death, he has found it challenging to meet with friends and attend social events in the village.

Scenario: Simon is in good physical health and does not require any support with daily activities. Having worked in a physically demanding job, since he retired, he has tried to keep active. Every morning he walks to the local newsagent to collect a newspaper and most days tries to work in his garden, although he feels much less motivated now that Annie is not there to share the activity with him. When Annie was alive, she did most of the cooking, and since her death, he has had to learn basic cooking skills. He is not very confident and eats simple food that he can buy in the village. He could drive to the supermarket in the nearby town but does not feel it is worth the effort just for himself. Simon also finds cooking a challenge and often he does not have a lot of appetite. He realises that some days the only interaction he has is with the newsagent when he collects his paper. He feels the emptiness of the house in which he and his wife shared so many happy memories. Sometimes he is overwhelmed by feelings of loss and sadness when he thinks about the future.

5.4 Mental Health

Simon visits his GP and says he is concerned about his lack of energy and reduced enjoyment of gardening. He is worried that these changes indicate the onset of a physical condition such as heart disease or Type 2 diabetes. In addition to a physical check-up, his GP asks Simon some questions about his appetite and activities, how much he is seeing friends and his social life. The GP reassures Simon that physically he is doing well. However, she suggests that he might have a depressed mood. His GP reassures Simon that how he is feeling is common after losing a spouse, especially when it is unexpected. The GP explains that men who live alone after the death of their spouse have an increased risk of depression in the first six months (Hung et al., 2021). This is also one of multiple factors identified as risk factors for loneliness in later life by the UK Campaign to End Loneliness (see Chap. 2: Table 2.1).

Simon assumed his lack of energy and enjoyment was due to a physical cause and did not consider a psychological cause. Depression is quite common in later life but is often undiagnosed (Allan et al., 2014). The World Health Organization reported in 2021, that 5.7% of the people aged over 60 across the world were experiencing depression (WHO, 2021). Whilst depression is more common in women, the risk of suicide, which is linked to depression, is higher in men, particularly as they age. Whilst globally the rate of suicide among 70+ older adults was 27.45 individuals per 100,000 (IHME, 2018), between 1990 and 2017 the rate among older men in the US was 48.7 individuals per 100,000 inhabitants and 140 individuals per 100,000 inhabitants among older men in rural China (Conejero et al., 2018). The US data are of particular note given that in 2019 older adults accounted for 16% of the US population but 19% of all deaths from suicide (ACL, 2020).

Among older adults, depression is often associated with other health conditions such as cancer and has also been found to be high in otolaryngology (ENT), dermatology and neurology outpatients (Wang et al., 2017). Taken with the increased suicide risk, there is a great need for services and solutions to address the mental health needs of individuals in later life. In many countries, government provided mental health services are commonly overstretched with long waiting lists. This has been heavily extended by the demands of COVID-19, both in terms of the impact of lockdown on people's mental health (Briggs et al., 2021) as well as the effects of long COVID (Naidu et al., 2021).

Simon's GP prescribes Mirtazapine, an anti-depressant drug, and also recommends he use a mood app to help him monitor his feelings daily and try to see if there is a pattern to when he feels better or worse. Although he is initially shocked at the diagnosis, Simon is also relieved to have validation that there is something wrong with him plus an explanation of why he is feeling this way. Following his GPs advice, he downloads Mood Kit and is surprised that he enjoys the daily journaling, as he has never written a diary or had any inclination to write about his feelings. He also appreciates the graphs the app produces which provide something visual for him to track. When he sees his GP again, he tells her that his mood has improved, and he is starting to engage in more activities in his community. He has heard about the local Men's Shed (see Chap. 11) in Desborough, a nearby town, and is looking forward to starting there and maybe picking up his carpentry skills again.

5.5 Technology Solutions

The development of technology solutions for late-life mental health has been increasing in recent years (Andrews et al., 2019). For example, data from sensors in everyday devices such as mobile phones have been proposed as one way to monitor mental health (Mohr et al., 2017). Attitudes towards using phones for monitoring depression, anxiety and stress are broadly accepted with appropriate safeguards for privacy (Proudfoot et al., 2010). In their study of older adult's attitudes towards using technology to manage their mental health, Andrews et al. (2019) found that interest was tempered by fear of the consequences of people, e.g., family or GPs, knowing they had low mood. A recent survey into the use of wearables to manage loneliness and social isolation identified four challenges: technological, socio-psychological, architectural and gerontological, relating to the digital ecosystem, physical environments, experience of loneliness and physical and health changes. Lack of knowledge of what technology and applications are available was also identified as a barrier (Site et al., 2022). The following sections introduce some of the most commonly available resources, highlighting those that have been developed and/or tested with older adults.

5.5.1 Mood Apps

The availability and use of mobile apps that promote positive mood and well-being have increased enormously in recent years. Among the most popular and widely known are Calm, Headspace, Happier, Mood Kit and MoodMission. For comparison, a brief review of their various attributes is presented in Table 5.3. Many of the current apps offer the popular mindfulness meditation which has been shown to improve mood. Others incorporate elements from Positive Psychology or Cognitive Behaviour Therapy (CBT: e.g., Mood-Hacker: Birney et al., 2016). Alternatively, clients undergoing CBT can interact with their therapists between sessions using an app (e.g., Giosan et al., 2017) (Image 5.2).

5.5.2 Technology for Social Isolation

Komp is a 'one button' computer that seeks to provide connections for those who are socially isolated and struggle with technology, whether through disability, inexperience, or lack of confidence. The computer is restricted to only delivering its core features:

Table 5.3 Functions of popular Mental Health and Well-being apps

Name	Variety of activities	User dashboard	Progress tracker	Onboarding quiz	Feedback	Group activities	Domain-specific content	Free	Research-based or app-tested
CALM[1]	Meditation		Basic stats	Yes			Guided meditation, sleep stories	To download but not to register	https://www.ncbi.nlm.nih.gov/pmc/articles/PMC6614998/
Headspace[2]	Meditation & mindfulness	Yes	Yes	Yes	Rewards	Yes	Music and sleep sounds	Yes, but limited—more features in the paid version	Studies available on the website: https://www.headspace.com/science/meditation-research
Happify[3]	Games & meditation	Yes	Yes	Yes	Score		Yes—tailored to the user	Yes—In-app purchases	Two published studies: https://www.ncbi.nlm.nih.gov/pmc/articles/PMC6996718/ https://mental.jmir.org/2021/2/e26617/
Mood Kit[4]	Activities & journal	Yes	Yes		Graph		Based on CBT[6]	No	Comparison study: https://www.ncbi.nlm.nih.gov/pmc/articles/PMC6582985/
Mood Mission[5]	Mental & physical	Yes	Yes		Score		Based on CBT[6]	No	Based on CBT research https://moodmission.com

[1]https://www.calm.com; [2]https://www.headspace.com; [3]https://www.happify.com; [4]https://www.thriveport.com/products/moodkit/; [5]https://moodmission.com; [6]CBT = Cognitive Behaviour Therapy

5.5 Technology Solutions

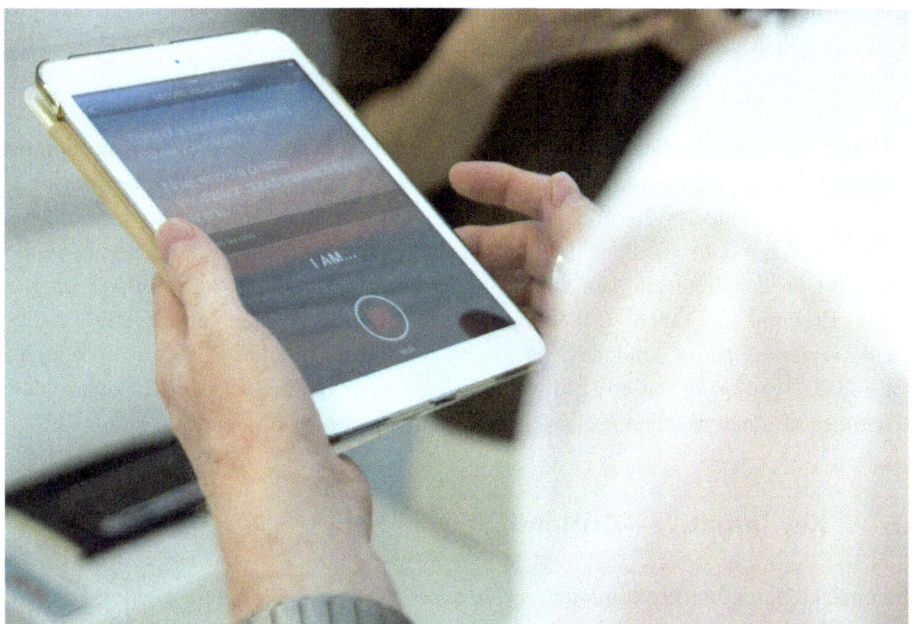

Image 5.2 *Credit* Simon Butler/University of Sheffield

photo-sharing, messaging, and video calling. Each of these activities is controlled by the user with a single button on the front of the device. Other design characteristics intended for simplicity include a non-touchscreen device, a large high-contrast screen, loud audio, and no requirement for usernames, passwords, or software updates. Komp was developed by No Isolation in Norway and is currently available in several European countries. In 2018 it won the Smart Aging Prize awarded by Nesta (a UK-based innovation agency), highlighting the most promising technological solutions in Europe that promote active aging.

5.5.3 Chatbots

As with the apps above, other technological innovations are based on existing therapeutic approaches for dealing with mental health issues. Bennion et al. (2020) compared two chatbots based on existing therapeutic approaches—Manage Your Life Online (MYLO)—which is based on a psychological therapy called 'method of levels'—where the therapist asks questions to help the client explore their own solutions (Mansell & Goldstein, 2020). The second was ELIZA, which uses a humanistic counselling approach to assist clients. Bennion and colleagues recruited 112 older adults to use MYLO or ELIZA and found lower problem distress at the end of the intervention for people who used MYLO. These users rated MYLO as more helpful, had longer interactions and were more likely to use it again than those who used ELIZA. These findings indicate the potential of online therapeutic interventions, whilst highlighting that different approaches may be more or less suitable for online delivery.

To facilitate direct contact, several similar services have developed in various countries to connect isolated people to local volunteers or workforces, who can provide well-being checks and assistance with simple tasks. These 'friendly visiting' services use mobile applications (apps) to facilitate connections, allowing users to make requests (either directly or on behalf of another person) and volunteers to sign up and help. Examples include Ensembl in France[1] Call&Check in Jersey[2] and onHand in the UK[3]. A systematic review is being conducted by researchers at the Belgian Red Cross (Laermans et al., 2020), exploring the effect of volunteer-friendly visiting services for older adults on feelings of loneliness and social isolation, as well as on well-being.

5.6 Key Initiative—OnHand

The onHand app connects community volunteers with people who are looking for companionship calls or support with daily tasks such as shopping or gardening. Older adults can make requests themselves using the app, or relatives, friends and carers can all access the service to post requests on another person's behalf. Non-digital users who wish to use the service can instead contact the organisers by phone to make alternative arrangements for getting their requests fulfilled. Funding for the service initially came from the charitable sector and is now provided by local companies who want to offer volunteering opportunities for their workforce. There is no cost to users for making requests or receiving visits. onHand has been evaluated by the National Innovation Centre for Ageing at Newcastle University in England, where the app has been trialled. The results, published in the company's Impact Report (2021), state that 60% of users wouldn't have asked for support if they hadn't used the onHand app, and that 90% reported feeling better than usual after having used it.

5.7 Find Out More

- The Centres for Disease Control and Prevention and the National Association of Chronic Disease Directors in the USA have produced this useful leaflet about mental health in later life: https://www.cdc.gov/aging/pdf/mental_health.pdf.

---

[1] https://www.ensembl.fr.
[2] https://www.callandcheck.com.
[3] https://www.beonhand.co.uk.

- The World Health Organization (WHO) produced this 2021 report about the impact of social isolation and loneliness on older people: https://www.who.int/teams/social-determinants-of-health/demographic-change-and-healthy-ageing/social-isolation-and-loneliness.
- Connect2Affect by the AARP Foundation (US) features digital resources aimed at reducing loneliness and social isolation among older adults. https://connect2affect.org/.

References

Administration for Community Living (ACL). (2020). 2019 Profile of Older Americans. Available at: https://acl.gov/sites/default/files/Aging%20and%20Disability%20in%20.America/ 2019 ProfileOlderAmericans508.pdf

Allan, C. E., Valakanova, V., & Ebmeier, K. (2014). Depression in older people is underdiagnosed. *The Practitioner, 258*, 19–22.

Andersson, L. (1998). Loneliness research and interventions: A Review of the Literature. *Ageing and Mental Health, 2*(4), 264–274.

Andrews, J., Brown, L. J., Hawley, M., Astell, A. J. (2019). Older adults' perspectives on using digital technology to maintain good mental health: Interactive group study. *Journal of Medical Internet Research, 21*(2), e11694. https://doi.org/10.2196/11694

Bennion, M. R., Hardy, G. E., Moore, R. K, Kellet, S., et al. (2020). Usability, acceptability, and effectiveness of web-based conversational agents to facilitate problem solving in older adults: Controlled study. *Journal of Medical Internet Research, 22*(5), e16794. https://doi.org/10.2196/16794

Birney, A. J., Gunn, R., Russell, J. K., & Ary, D. V. M. (2016). Mobile web app with email for adults to self-manage mild-to-moderate depression: Randomized Controlled Trial. *JMIR mHealth and uHealth, 4*(1), e8.

Briggs, R., McDowell, C. P., De Looze, C., Kenny, R. A., et al. (2021). Depressive symptoms among older adults pre and post-COVID–19 Pandemic. *Journal of American Medical Directors Association, 22*(11), 2251–2257.

Conejero, I., Olié, E., Courtet, P., & Calati, R. (2018). Suicide in older adults: Current perspectives. *Clinical Interventions in Aging, 13*, 691–699. https://doi.org/10.2147/CIA.S130670

Giosan, C., Cobeanu, O., Mogoaşe, C., Szentagotai, A., et al. (2017). Reducing depressive symptomatology with a smartphone app: Study protocol for a randomized, placebo-controlled trial. *Trials, 18*(1), 1–12. https://doi.org/10.1186/s13063-017-1960-1chat

Hung, Y. C., Chen, Y. H., Lee, M. C., & Yeh, C. J. (2021). Effect of spousal loss on depression in older adults: Impacts of time passing, living arrangement, and spouse's health status before death. *International Journal of Environmental Research and Public Health, 18*(24), 13032. https://doi.org/10.3390/ijerph182413032

Institute for Health Metrics and Evaluation (IHME). (2018). Findings from the Global Burden of Disease Study 2017. Seattle, WA. Available at: https://www.healthdata.org/sites/default/files/files/policy_report/2019/GBD_2017_Booklet.pdf

Laermans, J., Scheers, H., Vandekerckhove, P., & De Buck, E. (2020). PROTOCOL: Friendly visiting by a volunteer for reducing loneliness and social isolation in older adults. *Campbell Systematic Reviews, 16*(2), e1084. https://doi.org/10.1002/cl2.1084

Mansell, W., & Goldstein, D. (2020). Method of levels therapy. In W. Mansell (Ed.), *The interdisciplinary handbook of perceptual control theory: Living control systems IV*. Academic Press, pp. 503–515. https://doi.org/10.1016/B978-0-12-818948-1.00013-7

Mohr, D. C., Zhang, M., & Schueller, S. M. (2017). Personal sensing: Understanding mental health using ubiquitous sensors and machine learning. *Annual Review of Clinical Psychology,8* (13), 23–47. https://doi.org/10.1146/annurev-clinpsy-032816-044949

Naidu, S. B., Shah, A. J., Saigal, A., Smith, C., et al. (2021). The high mental health burden of "Long COVID" and its association with ongoing physical and respiratory symptoms in all adults discharged from hospital. *European Respiratory Journal, 57*, 2004364. https://doi.org/10.1183/13993003.04364-2020

National Innovation Centre for Ageing. (2021). OnHand—The Impact Report. Available from: https://www.uknica.co.uk/our-stories/onhand-the-impact-report/

Proudfoot, J. Parker, G. Hadzi Pavlovic, D. Manicavasagar, V. et al. (2010). Community attitudes to the appropriation of mobile phones for monitoring and managing depression, anxiety, and stress. *Journal of Medical Internet Research, 12*(5), e64. https://doi.org/10.2196/jmir.1475

Site, A., Lohan, E. S., Jolanki, O., Valkama, O., et al. (2022). Managing perceived loneliness and social isolation levels for older adults: A survey with focus on wearables-based solutions. *Sensors, 22*(3), 1–45. https://doi.org/10.3390/s22031108

Townsend, P. (1957). *The family life of old people: An inquiry in east*. Harmondsworth, Penguin.

Townsend, P. (1973). *The social minority*. Allen Lane.

Wang, J. Wu, X. Lai, W. Long, E. et al. (2017). Prevalence of depression and depressive symptoms among outpatients: A systematic review and meta-analysis. *BMJ Open,* e017173. https://doi.org/10.1136/bmjopen-2017-017173

World Health Organization (WHO). (2021). Depression. Available at https://www.who.int/news-room/fact-sheets/detail/depression

Staying Connected to Recreation and Leisure 6

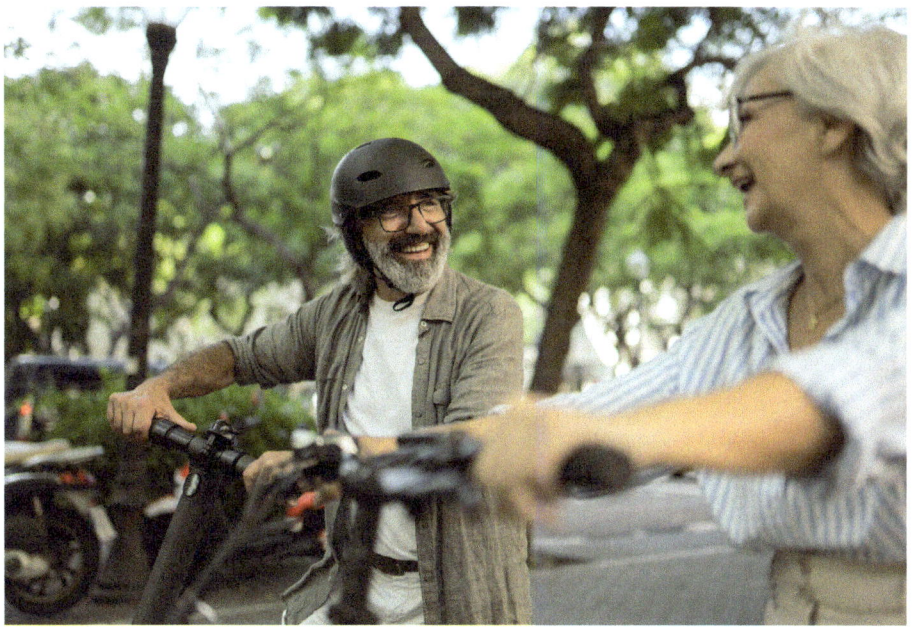

Image 6.1 *Credit* Shutterstock—PintoArt

6.1 The Challenge

This chapter is an accompaniment to the previous two chapters where we looked at the importance of social interaction for mental health and well-being, and the role that AgeTech can play. Such interactions can take place in multiple contexts and environments, adding to the benefits of social engagement. Many recreation and leisure activities, for example, take place in social settings such as groups, classes, teams, or congregations. These activities also provide opportunities to learn new skills or practise old ones, keep mentally and physically active, as well as making new friends or meeting old ones. Recreation and leisure activities in later life are particularly important for helping people adjust to life after paid work (Image 6.1). Having regular commitments to meet others for socializing, playing sports, or at a place of worship, for example, provides structure which is important for maintaining a sense of purpose. As with all aspects of daily life, technology is increasingly playing a role in how we access recreation and leisure activities.

6.2 What's in This Chapter?

In this chapter, we consider examples of technologies that support different types of leisure and recreation. Some of these use technology as a mediator or gateway to an activity, such as remote choirs or museum tours. The scope includes physical activities, artistic and creative pursuits, and of course, social interaction. Some activities are free to use. However, they still rely on individuals having access to technology to connect them to recreation and leisure activities—this point is picked up in Chap. 10 where we look at policy.

6.3 Persona and Scenario: Mathilde

Persona: Mathilde is an 80-year-old woman living in Rotterdam. She is single and worked as a nurse in acute medicine until she retired and now receives a state pension plus an occupational pension. She has always kept physically active, cycling to and from work every day. Living alone she has always enjoyed a busy social life, regularly attending theatre and opera with her friends as well as regular trips to the many local art galleries and those farther afield. Since finishing paid work, these activities have occupied more of her time. Every day she cycles to the local shopping precinct to meet friends for coffee and plan outings to local attractions or further afield to Amsterdam or Eindhoven.

Scenario: While cycling home from coffee one morning, Mathilde is in a road accident in which she breaks her dominant wrist, injures her shoulder, and suffers an orbital fracture. She is in hospital for one night where a physiotherapist starts active rehabilitation immediately after surgery. Shortly before discharge an occupational therapist (OT)

6.3 Persona and Scenario: Mathilde

comes to assess whether Mathilde will have any problems with everyday activities when she goes home. The OT says that she will organize a few basic assistive devices for Mathilde from the local homecare organization, to support independent meal preparation and safe mobility. At discharge, the physiotherapist advises Mathilde to continue rehabilitation with a local physiotherapist and provides written advice about further training. A few days after discharge the general practitioner invites Mathilde for a visit. During this visit, the GP discusses the rehabilitation approach and checks whether she has obtained the recommended assistive devices and whether these are effective. The GP also discusses longer-term possibilities for rehabilitation, including low-intensity physical activities such as walking, which Mathilde could access through a local club.

Although she has been told that she should make a good recovery, the accident has had a big impact on Mathilde. Having her arm in a sling means she cannot cycle. She is also feeling very tired, which she attributes to the pain medication she is taking, but it prevents her from being able to walk to meet her friends. One friend with a car has offered to come and pick her up for coffee but she is self-conscious of her facial injury which will take several weeks to fully heal and does not want to go out in public. At home, Mathilde tries to pass the time by reading but is finding it difficult to concentrate. This adds to her worries that she may have injured her head more seriously than she realised. She has always been proudly independent and does not like to consider that she may need assistance in the future as a result of her accident.

Solution: virtual tours

Mathilde owns a tablet, and her friend Yvonne tells her that many museums and art galleries in Rotterdam and across the Netherlands are offering online tours and activities. Mathilde has always enjoyed visiting the Maritime Museum and so she signed up to listen to the audio tours where employees describe their favourite objects from the collection. She and Yvonne also signed up for the Deshima Experience created by the Wereldmuseum. This is an interactive program exploring the story behind a Japanese screen in the museum.[1] Mathilde and Yvonne also explore the artworks and take virtual tours of the van Gogh Museum.[2] At the Rijks Museum, they enjoy putting together their own exhibit and exploring Rembrandt's Night Watch.[3] Taking the virtual tours alone or with Yvonne improves Mathilde's mood and she begins to feel more like her old self. As she recovers from her injuries, she starts to plan trips outside her home, using online tools to identify new places to visit with Yvonne and her other friends.

---

[1] https://www.volkenkunde.nl/en/deshima-experience.
[2] https://www.vangoghmuseum.nl/en/visit/enjoy-the-museum-from-home.
[3] https://www.rijksmuseum.nl/en/from-home.

6.4 Technology for Recreation and Leisure

6.4.1 Museums and Art Galleries

Many of the world's leading art galleries and museums offer virtual tours of their collections. The Joy of Museums website includes links to museums, art galleries and historic sites across the world.[4] The site includes curated tours such as Ancient Artefacts, Mythological Art, Famous Paintings, Christian Art and Biblical Paintings, Buddhist Art, and Famous Sculptures. The site can also be searched by continent, country, and city. For example, in Africa, the Egyptian Museum in Cairo has a tour of the Tutankhamun exhibit.[5]

Many world-famous museums and art galleries offer virtual tours and interactive activities, including those in London. The Natural History Museum has 12 virtual activities including a virtual self-guided tour of the galleries, an interactive experience about Hope the Blue Whale, and audio guides narrated by Sir David Attenborough. You can also meet the Museum's scientists and browse the archive.[6] At the Science Museum, you can explore the 325,000 individual items in the collection or take a virtual tour around the museum using Google Street View.[7] The British Museum has an interactive timeline for searching artefacts across history and the world,[8] while the Victoria and Albert Museum has an online program of events and activities for all ages.[9] The National Gallery hosts online events as well as virtual tours,[10] while the National Portrait Gallery has activities to do at home including Mindful Drawing and step-by-step guides to drawing and painting.[11]

The Google Arts and Culture app also provides access to multiple museums including the Guggenheim Museum in New York which uses street view for visitors to wander around the museum, and the Getty Museum in Los Angeles: find links here.[12] The National Gallery of Art in DC has two online exhibits one about Vermeere and the other about fashion.[13] Musée d'Orsay, Paris also has a walk-through tour for visitors.[14] The National Museum of Modern and Contemporary Art in Seoul has eight online accessible

---

[4] https://joyofmuseums.com.

[5] https://egymonuments.gov.eg/en/news/a-virtual-tour-through-the-tutankhamun-collection-at-the-egyptian-museum.

[6] https://www.nhm.ac.uk/visit/virtual-museum.html.

[7] https://www.sciencemuseum.org.uk/virtual-tour-science-museum.

[8] https://britishmuseum.withgoogle.com.

[9] https://www.vam.ac.uk/info/explore-the-va-online.

[10] https://www.nationalgallery.org.uk.

[11] https://www.npg.org.uk.

[12] https://artsandculture.google.com/?hl=en.

[13] https://artsandculture.google.com/partner/national-gallery-of-art-washington-dc?hl=en.

[14] https://artsandculture.google.com/partner/musee-dorsay-paris?hl=en.

6.4 Technology for Recreation and Leisure

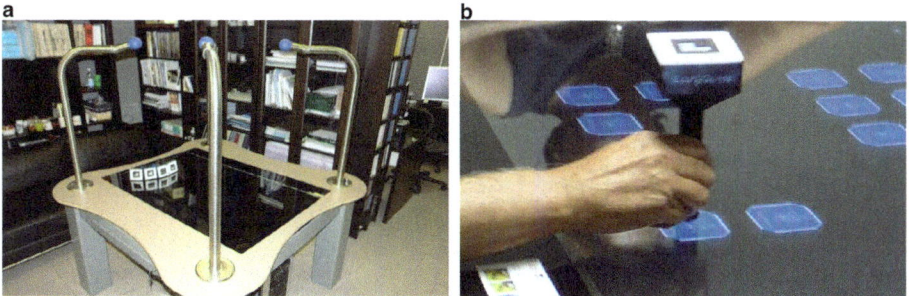

Image 6.2 **a** Eldergames interactive table. **b** Playing the memo game. *Credit* Gamberini et al. (2009)

through Google Arts and Culture.[15] These activities can be enjoyed alone or with others by providing access for people who are unable to travel. The activities can be used on a big screen in day programs and long-term care homes as well as by individuals in their own homes to explore with family or friends.

6.4.2 Digital Games

Another accessible recreational pastime is digital games. There are many free apps for people who have tablets or smartphones to use, as well as online games that can be played with others remotely (see also Chap. 7). Many computer games have an intrinsic social element, being played with one or more other people (Whitcomb, 1990). The Eldergames project, funded by the European Union, set out to use games as a medium for improving older people's quality of life. The team from Italy and Spain worked closely with older adults to create an interactive table for playing games with others (Image 6.2a, b; Gamberini et al., 2007). They examined participants' experiences along seven key dimensions which included: social interaction, playability/immersion, and challenge/skills. Overall, the participants reported that the biggest benefit of Eldergames was social interaction, defined in the study as the *'opportunity to create and maintain new relationships'* (Gamberini et al., 2009, p. 167). Sixty-six per cent of the participants endorsed the statement—*'The most interesting thing has been to share my time with other people while playing'*. This highlights the importance older adults attach to staying connected to others.

During the pandemic, opportunities for playing games in person were dramatically reduced due to lockdowns and quarantine. However, it is well established that the social benefits of playing computer games can also be delivered through playing remotely

---

[15] https://artsandculture.google.com/partner/national-museum-of-modern-and-contemporary-art-korea?hl=en.

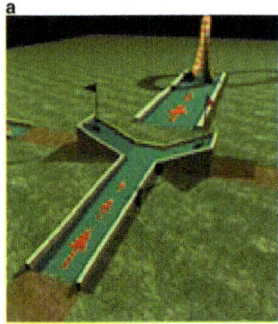 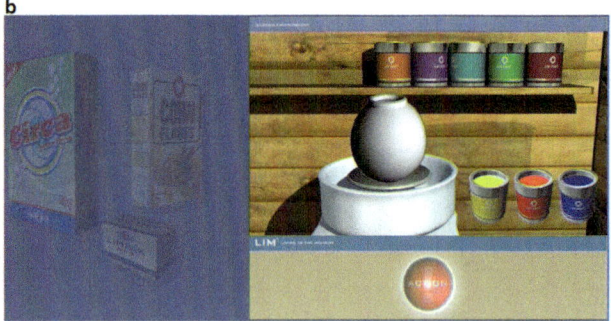

Image 6.3 **a** *Credit* Arlene Astell and LIM team. **b** *Credit* Arlene Astell and LIM team

(Astell, 2013). Long before the pandemic, research established the potential for exploiting the Internet for increased engagement and social interaction for older people, along with their willingness and interest to engage with technology. As with any other technology adoption decisions, older people are influenced by its potential for enhancing or increasing opportunities for social contacts, putting them in touch with people with similar interests, or enabling them to stay in touch with people when face-to-face interactions are not possible (Ijsselsteijn et al., 2007). This was ably demonstrated in 2009 by Khoo, Merritt and Cheok who created the Age Invaders System. Their system was designed specifically to facilitate intergenerational family entertainment with players, for example, grandparents and grandchildren in different locations.

With the advent of smart devices, including phones and tablets, access to games that can be enjoyed as a solo activity or with others increased enormously (Kaufman et al., 2020). In their white paper on gaming for older adults, Kaufman, and colleagues report on the multiple benefits of gaming including for mental and physical health, and well-being. They highlight that many older adults are playing games on their phones and as with the ElderGames project, they primarily value the social connectedness from playing with others. One challenge with smart devices is identifying games that are accessible (e.g., for sensory or cognitive impairment) and providing the right balance of challenge and reward.

As the ElderGames and Age Invaders examples highlight, research into digital games for older adults started long before smart devices were introduced. The Living in the Moment (LIM) project (2004–7) co-created and tested more than 30 potential games with people living with dementia (Astell et al., 2014). Many of these were rejected by people with dementia as unengaging, including crazy golf (Image 6.3a), whereas the painting game (Image 6.3b) was universally popular. LIM, which was created in Scotland, also included virtual tours of a house, a pub, plus the Botanical Gardens and McManus Gallery in Dundee, Scotland.

6.4 Technology for Recreation and Leisure

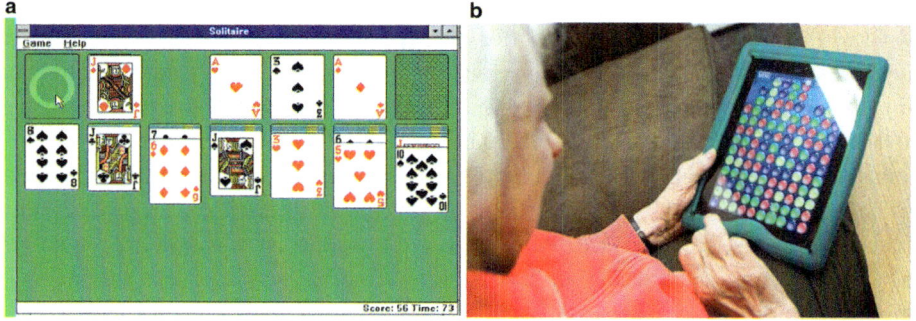

Image 6.4 **a** Solitaire. *Credit* Flickr. **b**: Playing BubbleXplode. *Credit* Simon Butler/University of Sheffield

Some of the research into gaming for later life has focused on serious games or exergames for physical and cognitive health (e.g. Baez et al., 2019; Boletsis & McCallum, 2016; See Chap. 7). However, there are millions of mainstream game apps in the Apple Store and Google Play store, many of which are free. With so many apps and versions of popular games, such as chess or Mahjong, it can be overwhelming to find suitable ones. The Accessible Touchscreens for Dementia (AcToDementia) project developed a framework to evaluate accessibility features of digital games for people living with cognitive impairment. However, these could be beneficial to anyone who wants to have more control over the games. Accessibility features include controlling sounds, i.e., turning them off if it is distracting or increasing the size of objects to make them easier to manipulate. The research team worked with two game studios to implement accessibility settings in one familiar game—Solitaire (Image 6.4a)—and one new game—Bubble Xplode (Image 6.4b; Joddrell & Astell, 2019).

Comparing the adapted versions to the originals, people living with dementia found the accessible version of Solitaire easier to navigate than the original. Bubble Xplode was easier to play in both versions, but participants in both groups experienced high levels of enjoyment playing both games. At the end of the project, both games were released by the studios with the new accessibility features. To assist people in finding accessible games, the AcToDementia website contains reviews of different games in English, Spanish and Mandarin. Suggestions for additional games to review are always welcome.[16]

6.4.3 Making Music

Listening to and playing musical instruments are popular leisure and recreation activities. These have long been recognised as an enjoyable pastime for older adults (Jansen & van

---

[16] https://www.actodementia.com.

Sadovsky, 2004). To facilitate engagement in musical activities, multiple projects have explored the potential of technologies for older people. A 2019 review of the research literature on using technologies to make music, confirmed that older adults are interested in engaging with music in different forms, even those with complex needs, for example, advanced dementia (Creech, 2019). A 2009 study developed ExPress Play, a prototype system for people living with dementia to create music. The system utilized chords to create pleasant-sounding music regardless of any prior musical knowledge, controlled through a touch screen interface (Reilly et al., 2009). Pilot testing with 10 people living with dementia found they were interested in using it, and identified adjustments to improve the usability (Reilly et al., 2009).

In a study at an adult day centre in a Hispanic community, Weisberger (2013) adopted GarageBand software to facilitate a songwriting group. GarageBand assisted the older people, which included individuals living with cognitive and physical impairments, to overcome challenges they experienced with acoustic instruments. Using GarageBand, the group created an album of 20 original songs. Weisberger (2013) suggested that GarageBand provided a framework for older people to explore tempo, rhythm, timbre, harmony, and melody and gain confidence in using a microphone.

Soundbeam[17] is an assistive digital music-making technology developed in the UK for use with children and adults, regardless of disabilities and impairment. To maximise accessibility, Soundbeam uses sensor technology to translate movement into music and sound, making it touch-free. The potential of Soundbeam for 'musicking' was explored in the AGE-WELL project, 'Promoting quality of life through creative and collaborative music-making with an assistive digital music technology'. A video about the project can be found here.[18] Other research into the impact of Soundbeam on older adults can be found here.[19] Music, Mind, Machine is a project in the UK which explored how new and emerging technologies can be harnessed for people living with dementia to enjoy music.

6.4.4 Singing

Like making music, the power of singing for delivering physical and mental health benefits is increasingly being recognised. A survey of 1124 choristers in England, Germany and Australia found that singing benefited well-being, particularly for women (Clift, 2010). A sub-analysis of the subjective accounts of 85 participants with high singing scores but low psychological well-being scores identified four categories of problems within this group: enduring mental health problems; family/relationship problems; physical health challenges and recent bereavement. From these accounts, the author proposed what they termed six 'generative mechanisms' that may account for the positive impact of

---

[17] https://www.soundbeam.co.uk.
[18] https://www.youtube.com/watch?v=vJlv6mjevOQ.
[19] https://www.soundbeam.co.uk/soundbeam-and-elderly.

singing on well-being: 'positive affect; focused attention; deep breathing; social support; cognitive stimulation and regular commitment' (Clift, 2010, p. 79).

Studies with older adults have reported a range of positive impacts of singing. An Iranian study with 60 older adults who attended a day centre, found that those who sang for 20 min twice a week for three weeks were significantly happier than the group who received care as usual (Entezari et al., 2019). The 'Community of Voices/Comunidad de Voces' trial in the US examined the impact of group singing on health, well-being, and healthcare costs (Johnson et al., 2020). Twelve, Administration-on-Aging-supported senior centers serving racial/ethnically diverse communities throughout San Francisco, CA, were randomized to receive the singing intervention immediately or after six months (wait-list control). The 390 older adults aged between 59 and 93 years of age (mean age 71.3), were drawn from four ethno-racial groups: Non-Latino white 34.44%, Non-Latino black 27.12%, Asian 202.9% and Latino 18.12%. Hypertension (52%) and arthritis (47.7%) were common among the participants, along with a range of other health conditions and 20% experienced financial hardship (Johnson et al., 2020. The main comparison carried out at 23 weeks found the singing group were significantly less lonely and had more interest in life after the intervention, but there was no change in the control group. During the project, health costs increased for both groups (doubled for the control group and tripled for the intervention group), but this difference was not statistically significant (Johnson et al., 2020).

A cost-effectiveness study in the UK calculated the cost of implementing and training staff to conduct singing groups over 12 months at £176.84 per session, at a total of £18.88 per participant over 14 sessions (Coulton et al., 2015). The study included 258 adults over 60-years-old randomized to a Silver Singing Group or control group. The singing groups participated in a 14-week 90-min programme comprising songs from different eras and a variety of genres. At three months there were improvements in mental health-related quality of life, anxiety, and depression, with maintained improvements in mental health-related quality of life at six months. As with the Community of Voices study, healthcare costs went up in both groups between the start of the study and six months later and were higher in the intervention group than the control but not significantly so (Coulton et al., 2015). They also calculated quality-adjusted life years (QUALYs), a measure of the state of health of a person or group in which the benefits, in terms of length of life, are adjusted to reflect the quality of life. One quality-adjusted life year (QALY) is equal to one year of life in perfect health. QALYs are calculated by estimating the years of life remaining for a patient following a particular treatment or intervention and weighting each year with a quality-of-life score (on a 0 to 1 scale) (National Institute for Health and Care Excellence, 2022). At the end of the intervention, the control group gained 0.008 QALYs compared with 0.023 QALYs in the intervention group, a significant difference (Coulton et al., 2015). Based on the outcomes of the Silver Singing groups study, Corvo et al., (2020) implemented the same intervention in Rome with similar results.

Singing for the Brain™ was launched by the Alzheimer's Society in 2003 to bring together people living with dementia, families, and caregivers to sing songs they know and love, in a fun and friendly environment. A qualitative evaluation of Singing for the Brain™ with 20 participants found they particularly valued the social inclusiveness of the groups (Osman et al., 2016). Other themes that emerged as important to participants were appreciating the shared experience, and the perceived positive impact on relationships and memory. They reported that attending the group lifted their spirits and assisted with acceptance of the diagnosis (Osman et al., 2016). The Alzheimer's Society also offers free resources for anyone wishing to set up a Singing for the Brain™ group.[20] In 2020 they expanded to offer 'Ring and Sing' for people to participate by video or telephone calls during the pandemic. As highlighted in Chap. 3, the pandemic led to a proliferation of virtual national choirs and singing groups.

6.5 Key Initiative—Art on the Brain

Participatory arts interventions such as expressive writing, creative storytelling, theatre, music-making, and dance, have been shown to positively impact a range of cognitive functions in older adults including problem-solving, memory, reaction time, as well as quality of life (Noice et al., 2014). In addition to providing choice and agency, arts interventions provide opportunities for social interaction with like-minded others. To bring participatory arts to older adults who struggle to access them, a team from Baycrest Health Sciences in Toronto, Ontario, led by Dr Kelly Murphy, developed ArtontheBrain (Murphy et al., 2021). ArtontheBrain engages participants in activities centred on user-selected visual artwork (such as a photograph, painting, sculpture, and/or textile. In a pilot study conducted with 31 older adults in Boston, Massachusetts, the art content available on the application was drawn from museum partners in Canada (Art Gallery of Ontario), the United States (Boston Museum of Fine Art), and open-source visual artwork material[21] and the artist Rafael Goldchain (Murphy et al., 2021).

ArtontheBrain comprises three functions: LEARN, PLAY, and MINGLE. LEARN provides the user with options to read (and/or listen to) the curatorial description of the artwork, magnify the artwork for closer viewing, or select to move on to another artwork; PLAY allows users to engage in puzzle games (involving three difficulty levels) such as restoring a visually scrambled image of the artwork. MINGLE allows them to share ratings of the artwork (using emojis), post comments, and view and comment on stories or comments shared by other participants. ArtontheBrain can connect people virtually to share their thoughts about an artwork in an online/virtual environment. The app has a tutorial video and gallery guide to provide instructions relating to the specific section the user is currently accessing. The 31 older adults accessed ArtontheBrain for 2 × 30 min

---

[20] https://www.alzheimers.org.uk/get-support/your-support-services/singing-for-the-brain#1.
[21] www.lacma.org.

per week, for 6 weeks. After the intervention the participants rated their interaction with ArtontheBrain positively, indicating they would continue using it and would recommend it to a friend (Murphy et al., 2021).[22]

6.6 Find Out More

- Chapter 6 of the World Happiness Report: "Social Connection and Well-being during COVID-19" describes the impact of isolation plus a helpful table of Protective Factors and Risk Factors for isolation having a negative impact: https://worldhappiness.report/ed/2021/social-connection-and-well-being-during-covid-19/.
- More information about the Community of Voices: https://cov.ucsf.edu/.
- A link to MusicMindMachine: https://mmm.sites.sheffield.ac.uk/our-projects/designing-new-musical-technologies-for-older-adults-wellbeing.

References

Astell, A. J. (2013). Technology and fun for a happy old age. In A. Sixsmith, & Gutman, G. (Eds.). *Technology for active aging.* Springer Science.

Astell, A. J., Alm, N., Dye, R., Gowans, G. M., et al. (2014). Digital video games for older people with cognitive impairment. ICCHP 14: *LNCS,* 8547, 264–271.

Baez, M., Nielek, R., Casati, F., & Wierzbicki, A. (2019). Technologies for promoting social participation in later life. In B. Neves, & F. Vetere, (Eds.) *Ageing and digital technology.* Springer.

Boletsis, C., & Mccallum, S. (2016). Smartkuber: A serious game for cognitive health screening of elderly players. *Games for Health Journal, 5*(4), 241–251.

Clift, S. (2010). The significance of choral singing for sustaining psychological wellbeing: Findings from a survey of choristers in England, Australia, and Germany. *Music Performance Research, 3*(1), 79–96.

Corvo, E., Skingley, A., & Clift, S. (2020). Community singing, wellbeing and older people: Implementing and evaluating an English singing for health intervention in Rome. *Perspectives in Public Health, 140*(5), 263–269.

Coulton, S., Clift, S., Skingley, A., & Rodriguez, J. (2015). Effectiveness and cost-effectiveness of community singing on mental health-related quality of life of older people: Randomised controlled trial. *The British Journal of Psychiatry, 207,* 250–255.

Creech, A. (2019). Using music technology creatively to enrich later-life: A literature review. *Frontiers in Psychology, 10* (117). https://doi.org/10.3389/fpsyg.2019.00117

Entezari, M., Zakizadeh, M., Yazdani, J., & Taraghi, Z. (2019). The effect of group singing on the happiness of older people. *Journal of Nursing and Midwifery Science, 6,* 78–83.

Gamberini, L., Alcaniz, M., Barresi, G., Fabregat, M., et al. (2007). Cognition, technology and games for the elderly: An introduction to ELDERGAMES Project. *PsychNology Journal, 4*(3), 285–308.

---

[22] Additional information about ArtontheBrain can be accessed at https://www.artonthebrain.org/.

Gamberini, L., Martino, F., Seraglia, B., Spagnolli, A., et al. (2009). Eldergames project: An innovative mixed reality table-top solution to preserve cognitive functions in elderly people. HSI 2009, Catania, Italy, May 21–23, 2009. https://doi.org/10.1109/HSI.2009.5090973

Ijsselsteijn, W. A., Nap, H. H., de Kort, Y. A. W., & Poels, K. (2007). Game design for elderly users. In: *Proceedings of the 2007 conference on Future Play, Toronto, Canada*, pp. 17–22. https://doi.org/10.1145/1328202.13282

Jansen, D. A., & von Sadovszky, V. (2004). Restorative activities of community-dwelling elders. *Western Journal of Nursing Research, 26*(4), 381–99.

Joddrell, P. M., & Astell, A. J. (2019). Implementing accessibility settings for people living with dementia in touchscreen apps. *Gerontology, 65*, 560–570.

Johnson, J. K., Stewart, A. L., Acree, M., Nápoles, A. M., et al. (2020). A community choir intervention to promote well-Being among diverse older adults: Results from the Community of Voices Trial. *The Journals of Gerontology: Series B, 75*(3), 549–559.

Kaufman, D. Sauvé, L., & Ireland, A. (2020). Playful aging: Digital games for older adults. A White Paper by the AGE-WELL 4.2 project. Available at https://agewell-nce.ca/wp-content/uploads/2020/02/AGE-WELL_WP4.2_White-paper_GAMES.pdf

Khoo, E. T., Merritt, T., & Cheok, A. D. (2009). Designing physical and social intergenerational family entertainment. *Interacting with Computers, 21*(1–2), 76–87.

Murphy, K. J., Swaminathan, S., Howard, E., Altschuler, A., et al. (2021). Accessible virtual arts recreation for wellbeing promotion in long-term care residents. *Journal of Applied Gerontology, 40*(5), 519–528.

National Institute of Health and Care Excellence. (2022). Quality adjusted life year. Available at https://www.nice.org.uk/glossary?letter=q

Noice, T. N., Noice, H., & Kramer, A. F. (2014). Participatory arts for older adults: A review of benefits and challenges. *The Gerontologist, 54*, 741–753.

Osman, S. E., Tischler, V., & Schneider, J. (2016). Singing for the Brain': A qualitative study exploring the health and well-being benefits of singing for people with dementia and their carers. *Dementia, 15*(6), 1326–1339.

Riley, P., Alm, N., & Alan Newell, A. (2009). An interactive tool to promote musical creativity in people with dementia. *Computers in Human Behavior, 25*(3), 599–608.

Weisberger, A. (2013). Garageband as a digital co-facilitator: Creating and capturing moments with adults and elderly people with chronic health conditions. In W. L. Magee, (Ed.), *Music technology in therapeutic and health settings*. Jessica Kingsley Publishers, pp. 279–293.

Whitcomb, G. R. (1990). Computer games for the elderly. In *Proceedings of the conference on computers and the quality of life*, Washington DC, US, September 13–16, pp. 112–115.

Staying Connected for Cognitive Stimulation 7

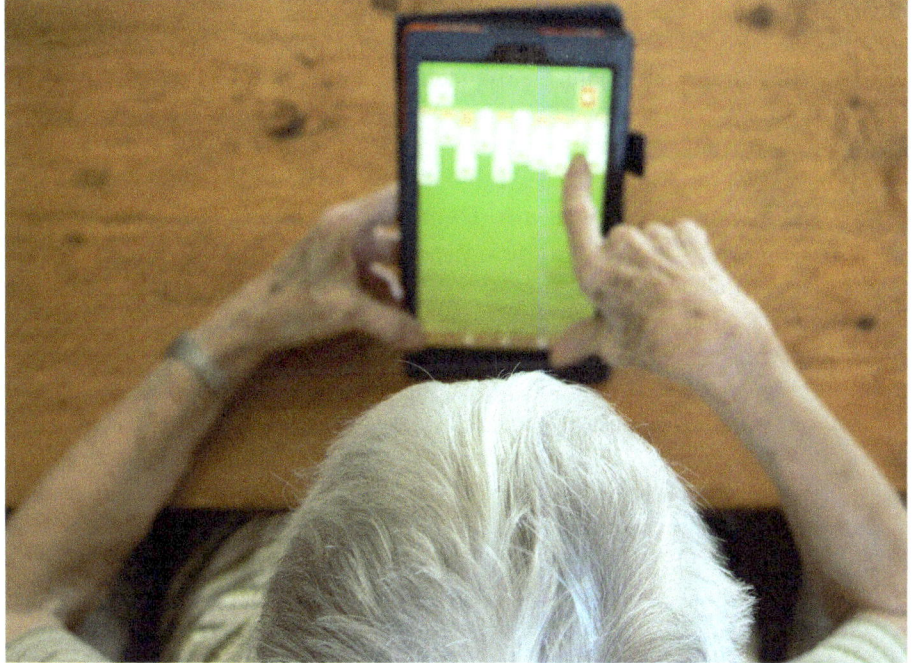

Image 7.1 *Credit* Shutterstock—Teresa Otto

7.1 The Challenge

There is growing interest in cognitive stimulation and staying mentally active as we get older (Image 7.1). In part, this is fuelled by fears about dementia, a condition characterised by progressive cognitive decline. Age is the biggest risk factor for developing dementia and understandably, the idea of improving or maintaining cognitive function has attracted global attention. Modifiable risk factors are aspects of lifestyle that can reduce the risk of various conditions. Interest in lifestyle interventions to reduce dementia was first suggested in the 1990s and has gained momentum across the world. Among these, social contact, connectedness, and social networks have been investigated as potentially modifiable dementia risk factors.

The purpose of identifying modifiable lifestyle factors is to develop interventions to lower an individual's risk. There is growing consensus that social interaction is one of the modifiable risk factors. Various bodies including the US National Institute on Aging (2017) and the Lancet Commission (Livingston et al., 2020) have produced lists of modifiable lifestyle factors. Probably the most comprehensive is the Lancet Commission 2020 Report which comprises 12 modifiable risk factors at different life stages (see Image 7.2: Livingston et al., 2020).

7.1.1 Social Connectedness and Dementia

In the 1980s, Australian researchers reported that people living with dementia wished for more social interaction (Henderson et al., 1986). Subsequent research from Japan identified '*psychosocial inactivity*' as one of five significant lifestyle risk factors for developing Alzheimer's disease (Kondo et al., 1994). In 2000, Fratiglioni and colleagues reported findings from the Kungsholmen project, following a cohort of 1203 community-living older adults in Stockholm, Sweden for an average of three years (Fratiglioni et al., 2000). During the study, 176 (14.6%) received a dementia diagnosis. Using the information on the participant's social networks collected when they entered the study, they found that dementia risk increased by 1.5 for individuals living alone and those with no close ties (Fratiglioni et al., 2000). The 2012 AMSTEL cohort study conducted in the Netherlands over three years with 2173 community-living older adults, reported that feeling lonely rather than living alone predicted dementia (Holwerda et al., 2014).

7.1.2 Social Interventions for Cognition

The evidence for the protective effects of social activity has inspired social interventions to improve cognitive performance. For example, a three-month intervention for 235 community-living older adults (mean age 80), involved participation in either therapeutic

7.1 The Challenge

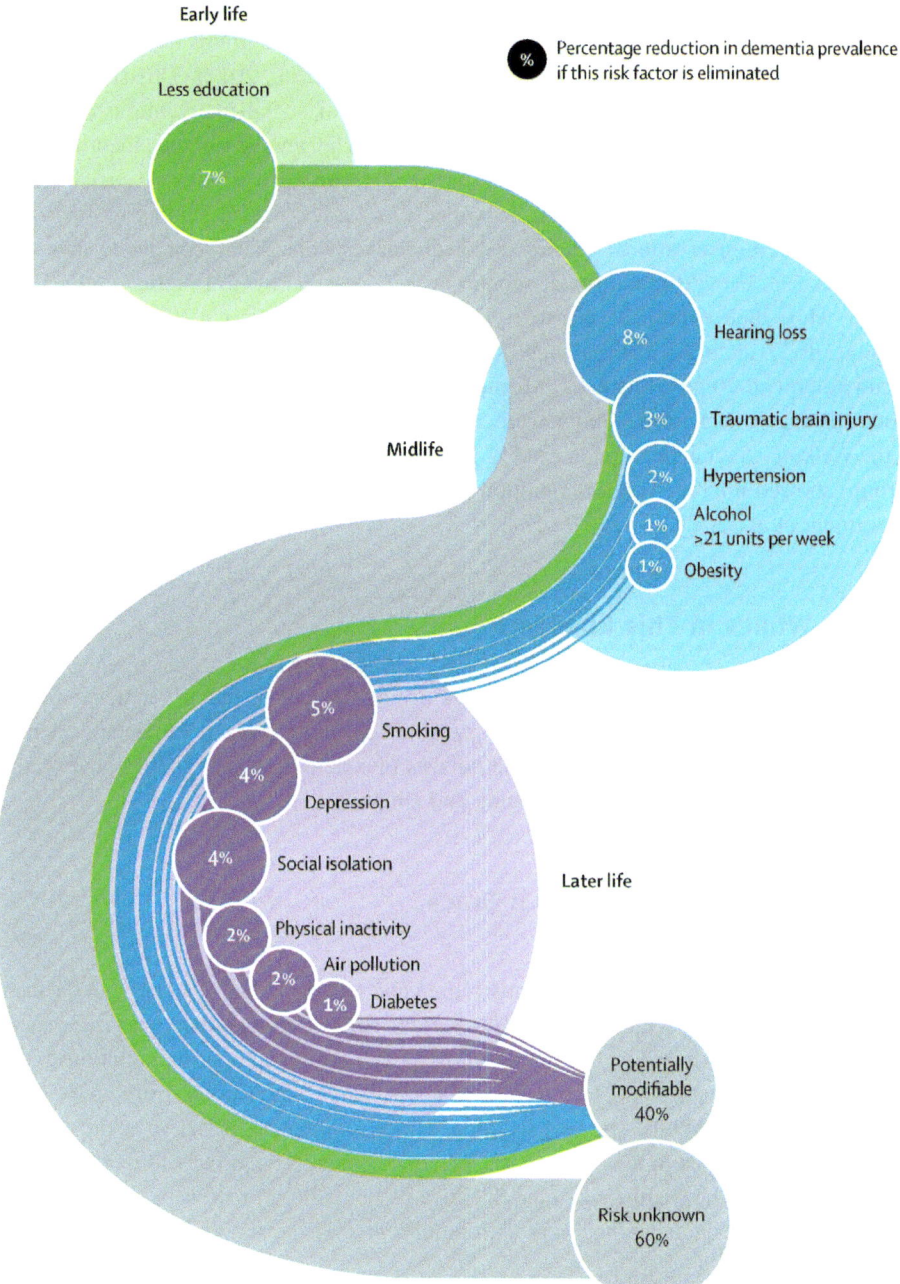

Image 7.2 Lancet 2020 12 modifiable dementia risk factors. *Credit* Livingston et al. (2020)

writing, exercise or art groups depending on personal preference. They found a significant improvement in cognition at three months in the intervention groups relative to controls, which was from the therapeutic writing groups (Pitkala et al., 2011). This study was one of three RCTs included in a 2017 systematic review of social interventions and cognition cited in the Lancet Commission 2020 report. The review authors identified three RCTs, 22 observational or longitudinal studies and two twin studies of social activity, nine observational studies of social networks, nine observational studies of social support, and three observational studies of social relationships. They concluded that social activity, social networks, and social support are all associated with benefits to global cognition, while their composite measure of social relationships, is not (Kelly et al., 2017). Another RCT included in the review looked at the impact of Tai Chi on cognition and brain volume at 20 and 40 weeks (Mortimer et al., 2012). One hundred and twenty older adults living in Shanghai, China were randomly assigned to one of four groups: Tai Chi, Walking, Social Interaction, and Control. Both the Tai Chi and Social Interaction groups showed improvement in cognition relative to controls plus increased brain volume (Mortimer et al., 2012).

7.2 What's in This Chapter?

Based on the evidence for social contact as a modifiable risk factor for dementia, this chapter looks are how technology can support social participation to maintain cognitive health. This includes online gaming and quizzes plus activities and other hobbies carried out in a group such as dominoes, dancing and singing.

7.3 Persona and Scenario: Grace

Persona: Grace is a 66-year-old, recently retired elementary school teacher from Clemson, South Carolina, in the United States. Her partner still works full-time, so Grace spends weekdays at home on her own. They recently moved to a neighbouring county to reduce her partner's commute, and Grace is now a couple of hours away from most of her friends and family. Whilst she was working, Grace maintained an active social life with colleagues and friends in the community. She enjoys exercise and likes to work out in the garden whenever the weather permits. She also uses a tablet to read news articles as well as listening to music and connecting with family.

Scenario: When Grace and her partner planned to move, they focused on finding a house they could be happy in that was close to local amenities. They are both concerned with sustainability and environmental issues and want to cut down on car usage, so they sold Grace's car when they moved. She can walk or take the transit to the local shopping centre and enjoys going out and about. However, since moving she often finds herself at a loose end and missing her social network from the old neighbourhood more than she anticipated. Grace had not given a lot of consideration to how she would fill the time that was previously kept busy with teaching and everything that goes along with it. Now she feels the days stretching out and is starting to feel lonely and somewhat isolated. Grace is also concerned that she is not using her brain as much as she did before. She is particularly concerned about Alzheimer's disease as she knows a few people in the community she used to see have developed dementia. She has found information on the Alzheimer's Association website about increased risk among African Americans and she wants to do things to help reduce her risk now she is not working. She realises how cognitively active she was when she was teaching. After so many years creating materials, planning, and delivering lessons and grading the children's work, she feels that her brain needs a workout. She is unsure where to start looking for something to pass the time, stimulate her brain and connect her with other people.

Solution: Online games

An old school friend who she keeps in contact with, tells Grace that she plays online games to keep mentally active. Her friend Ruth plays Lexulous, a free online word game that you can play with friends or make new friends. Ruth also sends Grace a link to the AARP website which has a list of recommended free games suitable for older adults.[1]

7.4 Technology for Social Connection and Cognitive Stimulation

7.4.1 Playing Games for Cognitive Stimulation

As discussed in Chap. 6, playing games can foster social interaction and engagement. Dominoes is a familiar game in many countries that provides both cognitive stimulation and social interaction. As a game with physical pieces, dominoes uses many cognitive skills including arithmetic, memory, tracking and planning to make moves. It is also highly social and can be played with a partner against another pair. Unsurprisingly dominoes have been investigated as a tool for teaching and learning. In his study of players at different ages—elementary school, high school, and adults—Nasir (2005) identifies several ways in which dominoes can be used in the classroom, including the relevance of the content and form of reasoning children were developing in dominoes to the knowledge they need in school. He also comments on the *'fluid coordination of individual cognitive activity and the structuring of social activity in the game of dominoes'* (p90), highlighting the dual benefits of cognition and social contact.

---

[1] https://guideforseniors.com/blog/senior-online-games/.

Domino players who develop dementia, have been found to retain detailed knowledge of the moves and gameplay in the face of declining cognitive skills (Greiner et al., 1997). Dominoes can be played online, and many online domino games exist. The Mexicantrain website contains seven domino games they recommend for older people to encourage 'dexterity, memory and social skills'. The first game, Mexican Train Dominoes is a free app described as simple to learn, that people can play with one or more other people online (see Sect. 7.6).

7.4.2 Group Activities

7.4.2.1 Exergames

Group activities can provide social and cognitive stimulation and also encourage physical activity. Engaging in physical activity has been shown to deliver many benefits in later life including neuroprotection (Mahalakshmi et al., 2020) and improved cognition (Erickson et al., 2019), as well as reducing fall risk (Sherrington et al., 2020). However, the majority of older adults do not meet the recommended targets for exercise per week (see the US Centers for Disease Control recommendations—Box 7.1). A large cross-sectional analysis of data from across Europe identified several reasons for inactivity, including increasing age, depression, physical limitations, and lack of social support (Gomes et al., 2017).

> **Box 7.1 CDC Guidance for Older Adult Physical Activity.**[2]
>
> Adults aged 65 and older need:
>
> - At least **150 minutes a week** (for example, 30 minutes a day, five days a week) of **moderate intensity activity** such as brisk walking. Or they need 75 minutes a week of **vigorous-intensity activity** such as hiking, jogging, or running.
> - At least **two days a week** of activities that **strengthen muscles**.
> - Activities to **improve balance** such as standing on one foot about three days a week.

A range of technology exists to promote physical activity and social interaction. Technology-based home fitness originally emerged in the 1980s with early exergaming platforms such as Dance Revolution (DDR; Konami Holdings) which transferred from the arcade to home on PlayStation in 1998. DDR players standing on a 'dance platform' receive musical (auditory) and visual cues to hit coloured arrows in a particular sequence. The arrows scroll up the screen and the player receives feedback on their accuracy allowing individuals to play against themselves or other players. The possible health benefits of

---

[2] https://www.cdc.gov/physicalactivity/basics/older_adults/index.htm.

DDR were quickly seized on with studies demonstrating the benefits of DDR on BMI and cardiorespiratory fitness of sedentary adults, obesity in children, and providing physical therapy for people with Huntington's disease.

Key to advancing exercise outside the gym has been developments in input technology. The first device using computer vision and gesture recognition to detect the user's movements was the Eye-Toy (released in 2003). This stationary webcam required the user to be within the frame for their movements to be detected. The Kinect substantially advanced gesture control with the inclusion of a depth sensor to detect distance and movement as well as four microphones to calculate the direction the voice is coming from. The Kinect also has voice recognition capability to aid in identifying which player is speaking. The home exercise genre became well-established with the launch of the Wii (2006) and Xbox Kinect (2010) home gaming systems. In addition to the home fitness market, both the Wii and Xbox have been widely adopted in healthcare for rehabilitation (e.g., Chanpimol et al., 2017) and physical therapy (e.g., Alves et al., 2018). For older adults in particular exercising with others rather than individually can lead to better participation (Silveira et al., 2013).

Baez et al. (2019) developed Gymcentral, a platform plus tablet-based fitness environment designed for independent-living older adults to keep physically and socially active. Older adults use Gymcentral in their own homes by joining a virtual environment which offers personalised training and feedback in a social setting. It has been designed so that *'members can interact and participate in group exercise sessions even if they have different physical abilities'* (Baez et al., 2019, p4). People living with dementia can also learn to play and benefit from exergames, particularly using motion-based technologies (Dove & Astell, 2017). There is evidence of learning as well as social benefits. When played in a group, people with dementia need fewer prompts, play faster, and take more independent turns (Dove & Astell, 2019).

7.4.2.2 Digital Cycling

Cycling has been shown to provide benefits to mental well-being and cognitive function of older people but can be a challenging activity to maintain. Electric bicycles (e-bikes) - bikes fitted with an electric motor that assists with pedalling—have opened up the potential for older people to keep or take up cycling. In their study comparing pedal cycles with e-bikes and non-cycling controls, Leyland, and colleagues (Leyland et al., 2019) found improvements in executive functions in both cycle groups plus improved mood in the e-bike group. A separate analysis of the participant's diaries kept during the eight-week intervention (Spencer et al., 2019) identified that while cycling, in general, encourages 'micro-adventures', e-bikes are particularly good for empowering people to connect with places and with other people. Spencer and colleagues concluded that e-bikes permit people to go further and provide confidence that they can get back home.

Spinning is an alternate form of cycling undertaken on a fixed bicycle. Spinning classes, where people cycle together guided by an instructor, are a popular low-impact cardiovascular workout. A variant is virtual cycling whereby the fixed bicycle is set up in front of a screen, so that riders can follow different cycle routes and join other riders, to simulate outdoor cycling. Cycling against on-screen competitors has been shown to increase the cycling intensity of competitive older adults (Anderson-Hanley et al., 2011).

Schikhof and Wauben (2016) explored a virtual cycling activity for people living with dementia as a means to promote and encourage continued cycling in a country where 36% of the population report cycling as their most frequent form of transport. Using a virtual cycling set-up provided by a Dutch start-up company (Wiltraco), Schikhof and Wauben compared the response of people with dementia to cycle routes and personalized images depending on interests. In this pilot study, eight participants aged between 60 and 93 (mean age 82 years) were observed as they cycled. They found that both conditions encouraged cycling, with the cycle routes slightly better at fostering engagement whilst personal images improved mood. Whilst there was no difference in cycling tempo, the personal images elicited much more discussion and interaction, which continued after the cycling ended.

7.4.2.3 Reminiscing

Another popular activity for groups or one-to-one interaction is reminiscing. Sharing stories is a way to connect with others and occurs throughout the lifespan (Fels & Astell, 2011). Telling stories develops early in life and is a social activity that occurs across cultures. Autobiographical stories or personal narratives are the substance of reminiscing. As demonstrated in Chap. 4, one approach to reminiscing is digital storytelling, to leave a legacy and promote intergenerational cultural transmission (Hausknecht et al., 2021) (Image 7.3).

Other technological approaches encourage reminiscing as a social activity, to promote conversation and build or maintain relationships. This is particularly important for people living with dementia, who find it difficult to speak about current events, leading to a loss of confidence in social situations. However, people with Alzheimer's disease retain the ability to recall and share stories from earlier in their lives and this can provide benefits in three areas—social interaction, maintenance of social and cognitive skills and presentation of the self as an equal conversation partner (Astell et al., 2010a).

The Computer Interactive Reminiscing and Conversation Aid (CIRCA: Alm et al., 2004) was developed to facilitate one-to-one or group reminiscing for people living with dementia and caregivers. CIRCA comprises a multimedia database of photographs, video clips and music to spark memories that can form the basis of conversation. Not only does using CIRCA support caregiving relationships (Astell et al., 2010b), a group study with 133 people, demonstrated significant improvements in cognition and quality of life (Astell et al., 2018). Originally developed in the UK, CIRCA has been tested in Japan, the Netherlands and Spain, and a Swedish version was launched in September 2020. A Canadian

7.5 Key Initiative—Dancing to Improve Health and Stay Connected

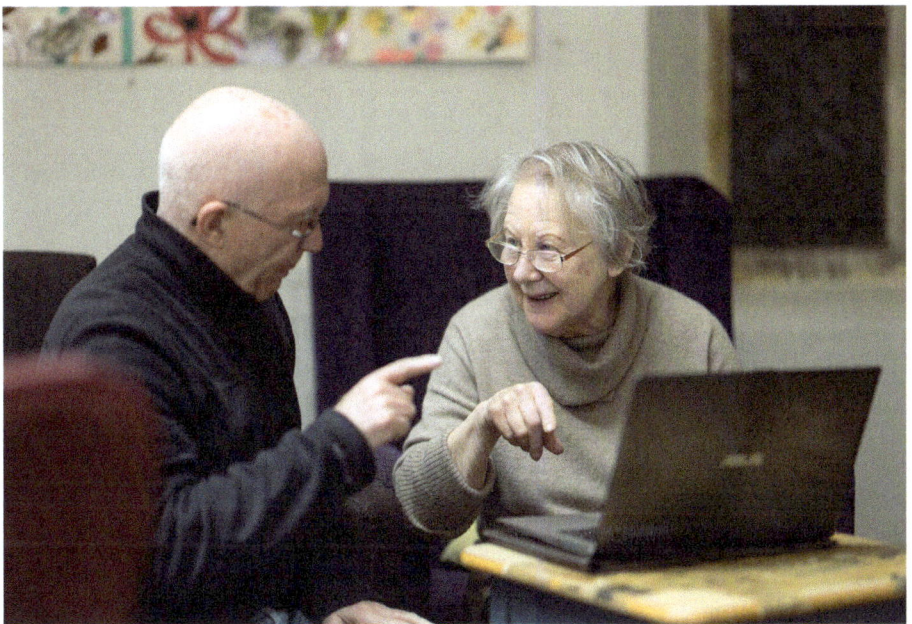

Image 7.3 *Credit* In-press photography/ageing better

version—CIRCA-CA—is currently undergoing community testing and a Chinese prototype was feasibility tested during the COVID-19 pandemic (for more information please contact Arlene Astell).

7.5 Key Initiative—Dancing to Improve Health and Stay Connected

In their 2021 book, "Dancing is the best medicine: the science of how moving to the beat is good for the body, brain and soul" Julia Christensen and Dong-Seon Chang, synthesise the evidence for the multiple benefits of dance (Christensen & Chang 2021). Not only is it a great form of exercise, with benefits for heart health, it provides social contact and can reduce stress. Research focusing specifically on the benefits of dance for older adults has demonstrated improvements in memory and attention in people with mild cognitive impairment (Liu et al., 2021), improved mood in hospital patients (Bungay et al., 2020) and reduced fall risk (Sherrington et al., 2020).

As already discussed, the COVID-19 lockdowns stimulated many services and activities to move online. In Hamilton, Ontario the GERAS Centre for Aging Research (GERAS Centre) at McMaster University and Hamilton Health Sciences responded by adapting their programs to online delivery. Their GERAS DANcing for Cognition and Exercise

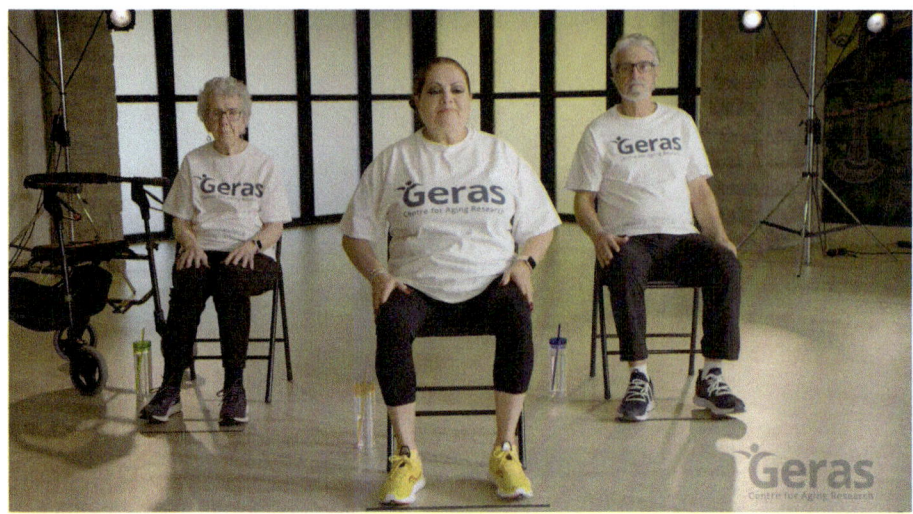

Image 7.4 GERAS DANCE for brain health and mobility: *Credit* Geras Centre for Aging Research

(DANCE) is an evidence-based and clinically proven mind–body health of seniors in the community with in-person and virtual programming (Hewston et al., 2022) (Image 7.4). Over the past 4-years, GERAS DANCE has grown from an idea to commercialization with prototype validation in 500+ seniors across 12 YMCA sites across Ontario. With AGE-WELL Strategic Investment Program funding, Dr. Patricia Hewston (AGE-WELL HQP) and team created an online community of learning to ensure program fidelity including standardized training and program delivery with interactive modules: our story, our population, our formula, our research, dancing in-studio, dancing at-home, new site bundle and instructor network. Virtual GERAS DANCE classes were highly successful in supporting seniors during COVID-19 to stay connected, building the LiveWell@Home Series: a partnership between the YMCA, GERAS, Hamilton Health Sciences and McMaster University (see Box 7.2).

> **Box 7.2: Dance Is Not Only Good for Your Body, Its Good for Your Brain!**
> GERAS DANCE is an evidence-based rehabilitation program for older adults who want to improve their brain health and mobility. It was developed with geriatric medicine and rehabilitation expertise at the Geras Centre for Aging Research, a joint research centre of McMaster University and Hamilton Health Sciences (HHS), partnered with the YMCA of Hamilton Burlington Brantford.
>
> Rehabilitation services are costly and of limited access or duration; alternative evidence-based options are important for older adults to prevent and treat frailty.

> GERAS DANCE is poised to become a signature rehabilitation program known for research excellence and unwavering commitment to improve the lives of older adults. By combining scientific rigour and the joy of dance, their mission is to transform the lives of older adults and make a positive impact both in Canada and globally.

7.6 Find Out More

- Mexican Train Dominoes and other domino games: https://mexicantrain.com/blog/seven-best-domino-games.html
- To find out more about GERAS DANCE and LIVEWELL AT HOME program, please email info@gerascentre.ca
- More information and resources for setting up and running Xbox Kinect bowling can be found on the Dementia Aging Technology Engagement (DATE) lab website: https://www.date-lab.com/.

References

Alm, N., Astell, A., Ellis, M., Dye, R., et al. (2004). A cognitive prosthesis and communication support for people with dementia. *Neuropsychological Rehabilitation, 14*(1–2), 117–134.

Alves, M. L. M., Mesquita, B. S., Morais, W. S., Leal, J. C., et al. (2018). Nintendo Wii^{TM} Versus Xbox Kinect^{TM} for assisting people with Parkinson's Disease. *Perceptual and Motor Skills, 125*(3), 546–565.

Anderson-Hanley, C., Snyder, A. L., Nimon, J. P., & Arciero, J. P. (2011). Social facilitation in virtual reality-enhanced exercise: Competitiveness moderates exercise effort on older adults. *Journal of Clinical Interventions in Aging, 6*, 275–280.

Astell, A. J., Ellis, M. P., Alm, N., Dye, R., et al. (2010). Stimulating people with dementia to reminisce using personal and generic photographs. *International Journal of Computers in Healthcare, 1*(2), 177–198.

Astell, A. J., Ellis, M. P., Bernardi, L., Alm, N., Dye, R., et al. (2010). Using a touch screen computer to support relationships between people with dementia and caregivers. *Interacting with Computers, 22*(4), 267–275.

Astell, A. J., Smith, S. K., Potter, S., & Preston-Jones, E. (2018). Computer interactive reminiscence and conversation aid groups—Delivering cognitive stimulation with technology. *Alzheimer's and Dementia: Translational Research and Clinical Interventions, 4*, 481–487.

Baez, M., Nielek, R., Casati, F., & Wierzbicki, A. (2019). Technologies for promoting social participation in later life. In B. Neves & F. Vetere (Eds.), *Ageing and Digital Technology*. Springer, Singapore.

Bungay, H., Hughes, S., Jacobs, C., & Zhang, J. (2020). *Dance for Health*: The impact of creative dance sessions on older people in an acute hospital setting. *Arts & Health, 14*(1), 1–13. https://doi.org/10.1080/17533015.2020.1725072

Chanpimol, S., Seamon, B., Hernandez, H., Harris-Love, M., et al. (2017). Using Xbox Kinect motion capture technology to improve clinical rehabilitation outcomes for balance and cardiovascular health in an individual with chronic TBI. *Archives of Physiotherapy, 7*(6). https://doi.org/10.1186/s40945-017-0033-9

Christensen, C. F., & Chang, D. S. (2021). *Dancing is the best medicine: The science of how moving to the beat is good for the body, brain and soul.* Greystone Books.

Dove, E., & Astell, A. J. (2017). The use of motion-based technology for people living with dementia or mild cognitive impairment: Literature review. *Journal of Medical Internet Research, 19*(1), e3. https://doi.org/10.2196/jmir.6518

Dove, E., & Astell, A. J. (2019). Kinect project: People with dementia learning to play group motion-based games. *Alzheimer's and Dementia: Translational Research and Clinical Interventions, 5,* 475–482.

Erickson, K. I., Hillman, C., Stillman, C. M., Ballard, R. M., et al. (2019). Physical activity, cognition, and brain outcomes: A review of the 2018 physical activity guidelines. *Medicine and Science in Sports and Exercise, 51*(6), 1242–1251. https://doi.org/10.1249/MSS.0000000000001936

Fels, D. I., & Astell, A. J. (2011). Storytelling as a model of conversation for people with dementia and caregivers. *American Journal of Alzheimer's Disease and Other Dementias, 26*(7), 535–541.

Fratiglioni, L., Wang, H.-X., Ericsson, K., Mayton, M., et al. (2000). Influence of social network on occurrence of dementia: A community-based longitudinal study. *Lancet, 2000*(355), 1315–19.

Greiner, F., English, S., Dean, K., Olson, K. A., et al. (1997). Expression of game-related and generic knowledge by dementia patients who retain social skill at playing dominoes. *Neurology, 49*(2), 518–523. https://doi.org/10.1212/WNL.49.2.518

Gomes, M., Figueiredo, D., Teixeira, L., Poveda, V., et al. (2017). Physical inactivity among older adults across Europe based on the SHARE database. *Age and Ageing, 46*(1), 71–77.

Hausknecht, S., Freeman, S., Martin, J., Nash, C., et al. (2021). Sharing indigenous knowledge through intergenerational digital storytelling: Design of a workshop engaging Elders and youth, *Educational Gerontology, 47*(7), 285–296. https://doi.org/10.1080/03601277.2021.1927484

Henderson, A. S., Grayson, D. A., Scott, R., Wilson, J., et al. (1986). Social support, dementia and depression among the elderly living in the Hobart community. *Psychological Medicine, 16*(2), 379–90.

Hewston, P., Kennedy, C., Ioannidis, G., Merom, D., et al. (2022). Development of GERAS DANcing for cognition and exercise (DANCE): A feasibility study. *Pilot Feasibility Study, 8*(9). https://doi.org/10.1186/s40814-021-00956-3

Holwerda, T. J., Deeg, D. J., Beekman, A. T., van Tilburg, T. G., et al. (2014). Feelings of loneliness, but not social isolation, predict dementia onset: Results from the Amsterdam Study of the Elderly (AMSTEL). *Journal of Neurology, Neurosurgery and Psychiatry, 85*(2), 135–42.

Kelly, M. E., Duff, H., Kelly, S., McHugh-Power, J. E., et al. (2017). The impact of social activities, social networks, social support and social relationships on the cognitive functioning of healthy older adults: A systematic review. *Systematic Reviews, 6,* 259. https://doi.org/10.1186/s13643-017-0632-2

Kondo, K., Niino, M., & Shido, K. (1994). A case-control study of Alzheimer's disease in Japan–significance of lifestyles. *Dementia, 5*(6), 314–26.

Leyland, L. A., Spencer, B., Beale, N., Jones, T., et al. (2019). The effect of cycling on cognitive function and well-being in older adults. *PLoS ONE, 14*(2), e0211779. https://doi.org/10.1371/journal.pone.0211779

Liu, C., Su, M., Jiao, Y., Ji, Y., & Zhu, S. (2021). Effects of dance interventions on cognition, psycho-behavioral symptoms, motor functions, and quality of life in older adult patients with mild cognitive impairment: A meta-analysis and systematic review. *Frontiers in Aging Neuroscience.* https://doi.org/10.3389/fnagi.2021.706609

Livingston, G., et al. (2020). Dementia prevention, intervention, and care: 2020 report of the Lancet Commission. *The Lancet, 396*(10248), 413–446.

Mahalakshmi, B., Maurya, N., Lee, S. D., & Bharath Kumar, V. (2020). Possible neuroprotective mechanisms of physical exercise in neurodegeneration. *International Journal of Molecular Sciences, 21*(16), 5895. https://doi.org/10.3390/ijms21165895

Mortimer, J. A., Ding, D., Borenstein, A. R., DeCarli, C., et al. (2012). Changes in brain volume and cognition in a randomized trial of exercise and social interaction in a community-based sample of non-demented Chinese elders. *Journal of Alzheimer's Disease, 30*(4), 757–66.

Nasir, N. S. (2005). Individual cognitive structuring and the sociocultural context: Strategy shifts in the game of dominoes. *Journal of the Learning Sciences,* (14), 5–34. https://doi.org/10.1207/s15327809jls1401_2

Pitkala, K. H., Routasalo, P., Kautiainen, H., Sintonen, H., et al. (2011). Effects of socially stimulating group intervention on lonely, older people's cognition: A randomized, controlled trial. *The American Journal of Geriatric Psychiatry, 19*(7), 654–663.

Schikhof, Y., & Wauben, L. (2016). Two types of stimuli in virtual cycling for people with dementia. *Gerontechnology, 15*(Suppl), p163.

Sherrington, C., Fairhall, N., Kwok, W., Wallbank, G., et al. (2020). Evidence on physical activity and falls prevention for people aged 65+ years: systematic review to inform the WHO guidelines on physical activity and sedentary behaviour. *International Journal of Behavioral Nutrition and Physical Activity, 17*(144). https://doi.org/10.1186/s12966-020-01041-3

Silveira, P., van het Reve, E., Daniel, F., Casati, F., et al. (2013). Motivating and assisting physical exercise in independently living older adults: A pilot study. *International Journal of Medical Informatics, 82*(5), 325–334.

Spencer, B., Jones, T., Leyland, A., van Reekum, C., & Beale, N. (2019). 'Instead of "closing down" at our ages … we're thinking of exciting and challenging things to do': Older people's microadventures outdoors on (e-)bikes. *Journal of Adventure Education and Outdoor Learning, 19*(2), 124–139.

Staying Connected for Intimacy

8

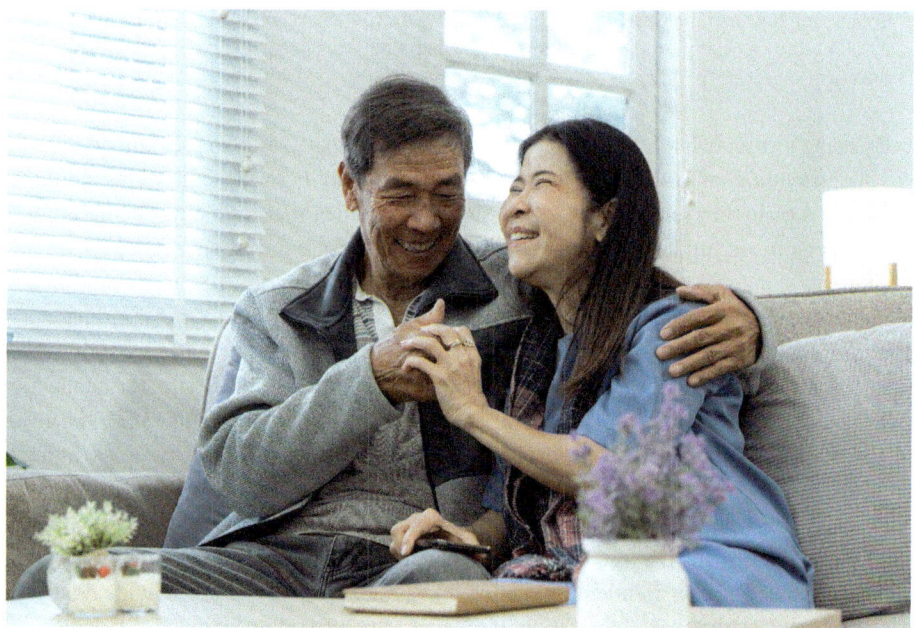

Image 8.1 *Credit* Shutterstock: Worawee Meepian

8.1 The Challenge

As stated in the previous chapters, staying connected to other people is a vital part of being a human (Image 8.1). One important part is intimacy, the experience of *'closeness, connectedness, and bondedness experienced in loving relationships'* (Sternberg, 1986). Fromm-Reichmann (1959) identified 'real' loneliness as the want of intimacy, which is different from solitude or the transient feelings when a person is simply left alone. Sullivan (1955) also argued that *'Loneliness… is the exceedingly unpleasant experience connected with inadequate discharge of the need for human intimacy, for interpersonal intimacy'* (p. 290). Intimacy can be defined as a close emotional attachment (Weiss, 1973) and occurs across the lifespan. For example, Zeedyk (2006) proposed that interactions between infants and parents, especially mothers, are *'undeniably intimate'*. She continues:

> Exchanges [between infant and parent] follow a reliable pattern of ascending and then descending levels of pleasure, in which the building excitement reaches an interim climax that is followed by a brief period of repose, during which time each partner can regain control over their arousal level. (p. 322)

By using terms such a 'pleasure ', 'arousal' and 'climax', Zeedyk is seeking to broaden our understanding of intimacy beyond sexual behaviour between consenting adults to other forms of loving relationships. This supports the idea that intimacy—being close to another person—is fundamental and is experienced across the lifespan.

A survey conducted by Ashely Macleod as part of her doctoral research found that as people grow older, sexual behaviour is still important to many, but for most intimacy and affection matter more (Macleod, 2020). Her work revealed that people especially value trust, respect, and compatibility as they get older, with an overall desire for connection with a partner. However, loss of intimacy in later life is common and there is growing concern that older people are excluded from having a valid identity as an intimate being (Simpson et al., 2017). This means the needs of older adults for intimacy are often overlooked, although this can have a profound effect on mental health and well-being.

Multiple reasons for the loss of intimacy have been proposed. In their study with older adults in assisted living, Bender, and colleagues (2020) found that an individual's health and functional status were barriers to intimacy. Other barriers included availability or access to partners, limited privacy and social rules and norms (Bender et al., 2020), which are not limited to assisted living. Exploration of intimacy in care homes reports similar obstacles, often intertwined with ethical challenges relating to residents with impaired cognition. Decisions about intimacy and sexuality in care settings are frequently made by staff without recourse to organizational policies or education on how to communicate with residents and their families about this topic (Cook et al., 2017). As a result, staff experience *'moral uncertainty and moral distress'*, often as a result of feeling more aware of residents' capabilities and wishes in terms of intimate relationships, than their family members (Cook et al., 2017).

Another important aspect of intimacy that is frequently lost in later life is touch, which delivers specific benefits from birth to the end of life. For example, in a recent study where some participants were touched but not others, the participants who experienced touch, reported lower loneliness scores, and this was more pronounced for single people (Heatley Tejada et al., 2020). The authors proposed that the availability of physical contact may help to explain the role of marriage as a protective factor against loneliness (see Chap. 5). Another benefit of touch in this study was a faster reduction in heart rate, which is taken as an indicator of physiological well-being (Heatley Tejada et al., 2020). Many older people experience loss of touch after the death of a partner or moving into a care setting, and despite the importance of touch for well-being (Field, 2010), this has received limited attention in service delivery.

8.2 What's in This Chapter?

As people age, opportunities for intimacy frequently reduce through ill health, physical or cognitive disability, bereavement, social isolation, or depression. This chapter explores a variety of ways in which AgeTech is tackling the need for intimacy in later life. We examine a range of technologies both general and specific, and services that can allow older adults to explore different aspects of intimacy. These include dating and sexual activity but also non-sexual physical and emotional intimacy. Technology considered includes dating apps, sex robots, and technologies delivering touch to those who seek it.

8.3 Persona and Scenario: Edwin

Persona: Edwin is a 75-year-old gay man living in Malmö, Sweden. He receives the national retirement pension plus a small occupational pension from his job as a draughtsman. Edwin contracted polio in his childhood and is now experiencing a range of physical changes associated with post-polio syndrome (PPS), which occurs in up to half of people who had childhood polio. After many years of stability, he has developed progressive weakness, fatigue, musculoskeletal pain, and muscular atrophy. People with PPS must avoid too much exertion and need to rest in between periods of physical activity. When he was first diagnosed with PPS, he was referred to a physiotherapist for low-intensity muscle-strengthening exercises, specially designed to be non-fatiguing. Initially, he was able to do the exercises daily but found he needed longer breaks in between to recover. Edwin was also referred to an Occupational Therapist who helped him identify ways to adapt his home and daily routine. As his mobility is affected, he currently uses a cane to help him get about. However, in future, he may need to use a mobility scooter or wheelchair.

Scenario: There is no cure for PPS and Edwin is concerned about his future and that of his partner. Until recently Edwin cared for Johan, his partner of 40 years, who was diagnosed with Alzheimer's disease five years ago. Over time Johan's cognitive status declined, and he relied more and more on Edwin to look after every aspect of their daily lives. As he needed to provide more physical care for Johan, Edwin found he had no energy left for exercising to help manage his PPS. With his physical deterioration, Edwin became unable to provide the care Johan required, and he moved into a care home five months ago. Edwin visits Johan every day for up to two hours but increasingly finds that he is exhausted for the rest of the day. With his days taken up visiting Johan and then recovering from the trip to the care home, Edwin finds he has no time or energy to meet with their small group of close friends. He misses Johan's presence and feels lonely in the apartment they shared for many years. Most of all he misses the closeness of sharing his life with another person, the brief touches, and hugs, and lying beside another person.

The solution: A friend who had gone through bereavement a few years earlier, tells Edwin about two devices that helped him through. The first was purchasing a smart speaker (as described in Chap. 3). The smart speaker provides the opportunity to hear a voice whenever the user chooses, which can provide comfort and a feeling of presence (Astell & Clayton, 2024). The second is InmuRelax,[1] a technology developed in Denmark that provides soft music and gentle vibrations to help the user fall asleep. The InmuRelax sensors detect interaction and breathing so it can detect when you fall asleep and stops the music. To date, small-scale research has demonstrated benefits from InmuRelax for different populations. Edwin is initially sceptical about both devices but with his friend's support tries them both. He finds the smart speaker becomes like a companion so that he does not feel he is coming back to an empty house. At bedtime, he finds that holding the InmuRelax not only helps him fall asleep but also provides a reassuring touch.

8.4 Technology for Intimacy

8.4.1 Hugging Technology

Various technological solutions have been explored to address the need for intimacy and touch, including several to simulate hugs. The Hug (DiSalvo et al., 2003) was an early concept for a robotic product to support 'intimate communication' over a distance. The development of the Hug was inspired by the team's research on aging to provide more accessible channels for intimate communication. In their research article, they present possible scenarios of use between Mary in Chicago and her granddaughter Chrissy in Pittsburgh sending 'messages' via the Hug.

---

[1] https://inmutouch.com/sleep/.

Other hugging prototypes include Hug over a Distance (Mulleler et al., 2005) a prototype device comprising an inflatable vest that could create the sensation of a hug when triggered and Huggy Pajama (Teh et al., 2008) another inflatable device developed for parents and children. HugMe (Cha et al., 2008) used a vibrating motor and HaptiHug (Tsetserukou, 2010) was a device comprising a belt and two soft hands that stretch around the chest of the user. Whilst none of these have progressed beyond the prototype or proof of concept stage, they do confirm the desire for touch remains strong.

One product that is available to purchase is Hug Shirt (Image 8.2; CuteCircuit, 2022).[2] Originally launched in 2002, its creators describe it as a *'shirt that makes people send hugs over a distance'*. The Hug Shirt was identified as one of the best inventions of 2006 by Time Magazine. Hug Shirt embeds sensors to detect touch and heartrate and connect via Bluetooth to any phone and can be purchased from its UK creators at CuteCircuit. According to the creators, during the pandemic, they delivered the shirts and its newest embodiment, the SoundShirt[3] to care homes and immunocompromised patients, and benefits were reported by the NHS. Angelini et al. (2014) also developed Hugginess, a prototype t-shirt with sensors and conductive fabric. Another prototype device using fabric was Keep in Touch (Motamedi, 2007). This 'networked fabric touchscreen is designed to support and maintain intimacy for couples in long-distance relationships' (p. 21). A blurred image of each partner was displayed on the fabric touchscreen, which came into focus as different parts were touched.

8.4.2 Online Relationships

Research has identified that a form of intimacy can occur in online relationships that are similar in meaning and stability to offline relationships (Lomanowska & Guitton, 2016). These authors also note that self-disclosure and social support—two key elements of intimacy—can provide positive psychosocial benefits when they occur in online relationships. Lomanowska and Guitton (2016) also consider how virtual reality and 3D avatars can create a sense of 'embodiment', which can enhance the experience of physical presence through haptic feedback (such as discussed in Sect. 8.4.1).

In terms of using the Internet to make new connections and relationships, older adults use it for similar reasons to younger ones. An early investigation by Adams et al. (2003) found that older adults were using chat rooms, dating sites, and online advertisements to try to find romantic partners. Romantic relationships that were formed online through dating sites or discussion groups, were intimate and long lasting (Malta, 2007). In her study, Malta also found that in addition to meeting romantic partners online, older adults (aged 61–85 years) were online flirting, whilst others used them to engage in extra-dyadic sexual relationships. The majority of participants in Malta's study were engaged in sexual

---

[2] https://cutecircuit.com/hugshirt/.
[3] https://cutecircuit.com/soundshirt/.

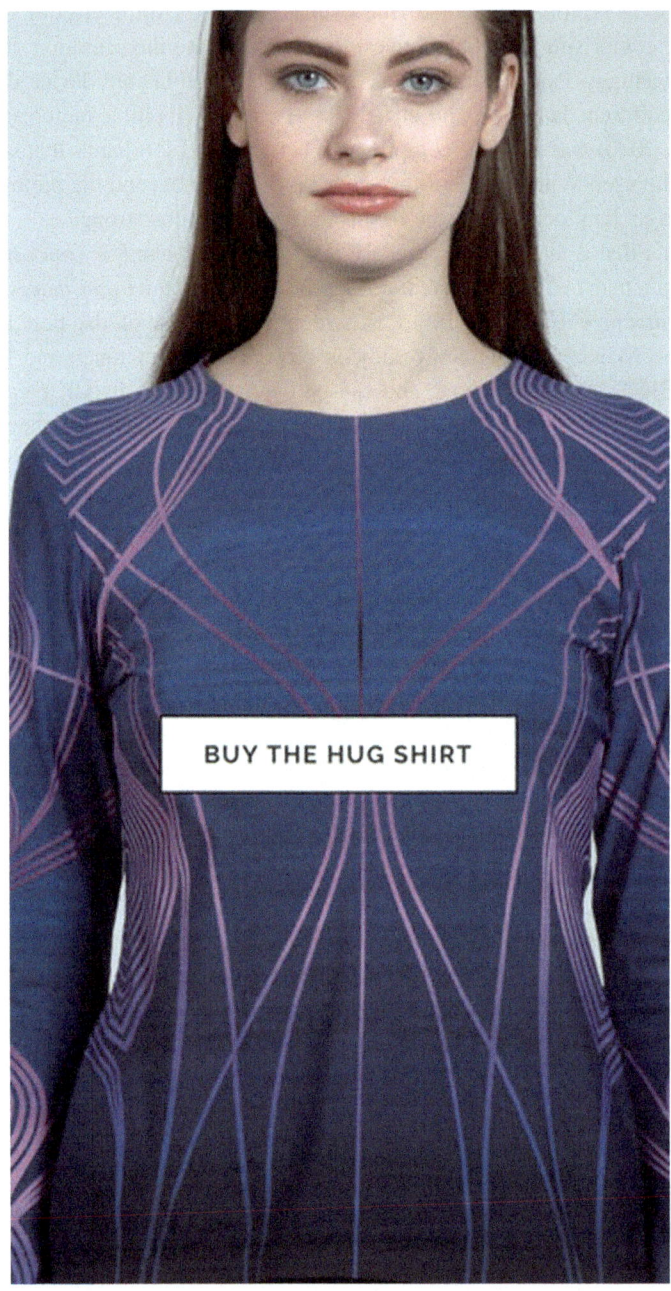

Image 8.2 *Credit* CuteCircuit

8.4 Technology for Intimacy

activity with the partners they met online, with some reporting cybersex had played a part in their relationships. Cybersex refers to a virtual sexual encounter where people send each other explicit messages describing a sexual experience, and may include masturbation (Malta, 2007).

More recent research has explored the occurrence of different types of online sexual activity identifying one category—partnered arousal activities—that relates to connecting with others (Scandurra et al., 2022). This can include engaging in webcam sex or sexual chat, activities which require a virtual interactive participation of at least two people. Another category—non-arousal activities—can include chatting on dating websites. A third category—solitary-arousal activities, relates to online activities such as watching pornography, which do not involve another person, and can damage intimacy in relationships (Minarcik et al., 2016). Concerning online sexual activities with others, Scandurra and colleagues (2022) found that 29.9% of their sample of 114 older Italian adults (aged 52–79 years) had engaged in partnered arousal activities 2 or 3 times in the previous month and 38.6% had engaged in non-arousal activities including chat rooms.

In December 2021, Forbes Health published its Guide to The Best Senior Dating Sites of 2022.[4] The article points to the health benefits of dating—including heart health and longevity—as well as what to expect and look out for if joining these websites. The article concludes with tips for safe dating and how to avoid dating scams. Sites such as Silver Singles[5] and Our Time[6] are aimed at over 50 s, whereas others such as Tinder[7] and Plenty of Fish[8] are general dating sites. Other sites aimed at over 50 s such as Stitch.net[9] and Amintro[10] are for companionship. Data released by Tinder for 2022 reveals that it has 75 million users, 78% are men, with 1% in the 55–64 age group (the oldest reported). The availability of sites specifically for over-50 s could reflect different motivations of older adults, or greater comfort with people at a similar life stage.

8.4.3 Technology for Sexual Activity

Regarding late-life intimacy through sexual activity, there is growing evidence of continued desire and interest, although there are also challenges and obstacles. Among those over 75, psychosocial barriers including stereotypes about aging, lack of partners and relationship issues have been identified (Garrett, 2014). Health-related barriers have also been reported. A study of sexual behaviour in 3343 older adults (55–74 years) in the UK,

---

[4] https://www.forbes.com/health/healthy-aging/best-senior-dating-sites/.
[5] https://www.silversingles.co.uk.
[6] https://www.ourtime.co.uk.
[7] https://tinder.com.
[8] https://www.pof.com.
[9] https://www.stitch.net.
[10] https://amintro.com.

found that 26.9% of men and 17.1% of women aged 55–74 reported having a health condition that affected their sex life (Erens et al., 2019). They found that individuals in close relationships made efforts to compensate for the impact of health problems, whereas ill health provided an excuse to stop sex or deter attempts to resolve difficulties in less close relationships.

To better understand health and other problems older people face in their sex lives, the Sexual Relations, and Activities Questionnaire (SRA-Q) was included in the English Longitudinal Study on Ageing (ELSA) of adults aged 50–90 years, in the sixth wave (2012–13). Questions in the SRA-Q relate to attitudes towards sex, current sexual relationships, frequency of sexual activities, difficulties with sexual activities, and concerns or worries about sexual activities (Hinchliff et al., 2018). 7079 completed the SAR-Q, of whom 1084 (680 women, 404 men) added additional comments. These 680 women had fewer lifetime partners, were less likely to have had sex in the previous 12 months and had more depression than the 404 men (Hinchliff et al., 2018). Analysis of the comments from these 1084 participants revealed that sexual difficulties negatively impacted psychological well-being although few people sought help for sexual problems. Where sex was uncommon or no longer happened, many relationships were still close and found other ways to share intimacy.

There has been limited exploration of technology to assist older people and people with disabilities to engage in sexual activity. One exception is IIS or Intimate Interface System for people with disabilities to explore cybersex in an inclusive manner (Fels et al., 2015). Comprising a virtual world with customizable avatars, animations and sound combined with a vibrating chair and pressure pad. The IIS leveraged the Emoti-Chair, a vibrotactile device, created by the first author's lab for deaf people to experience music (Karam et al., 2008). Early research revealed that when vibrations from the Emoti-Chair were applied to their bottom and genitalia, people felt excited (Fels et al., 2015). IIS was developed as an island with different locations (Image 8.3a–d) and participants were invited to explore different scenarios whilst sitting in or touching the Emoti-Chair. Outputs from the study included design recommendations for future iterations giving more control to people with disabilities and adding features such as temperature control and more realistic graphics (Fels et al., 2015).

Whilst IIS is a bespoke technology co-created with end users, sex robots are existing products, whose use by older adults and people with disabilities has started to be explored. In an attention-grabbing article entitled 'Nothing to be Ashamed of: Sex Robots for Older Adults with Disabilities', Jecker (2021) a professor in the Bioethics Department at the University of Washington, put forward an argument for access to sex robots for older people with disabilities. Jecker (2021) uses the description of sex robots provided by Gersen (2019) as…

> Life-size machine entities with human-like appearance, movement, and behaviour, designed to interact with people in erotic and romantic ways… with capabilities ranging from simple

8.4 Technology for Intimacy

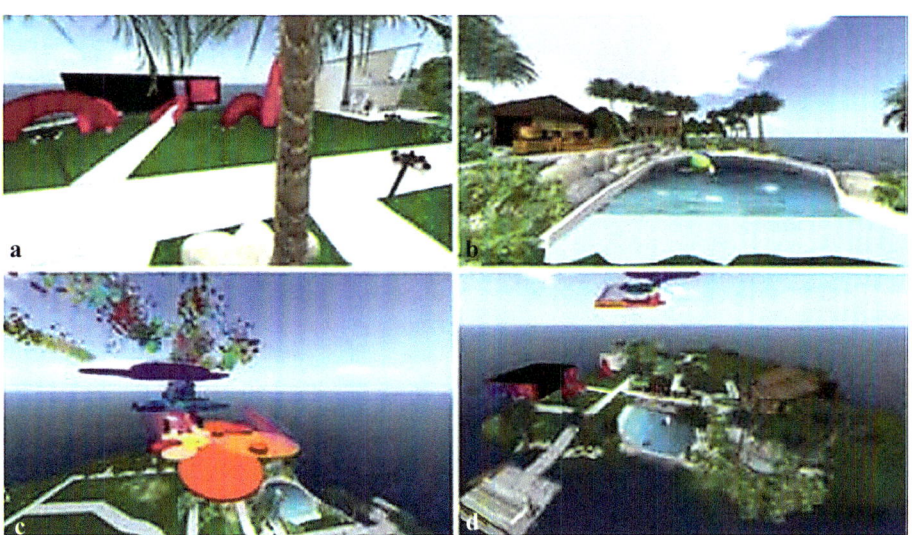

Image 8.3 **a** Night club and a private home with connecting brick pathways; **b** pool area with beach entry; **c** floating "hang-out" area; and **d** full island birds-eye view. *Credit* Fels et al. (2015)

> verbal responses to physical movements to more advanced artificial intelligence. (pp. 1794–95)

Basing her argument on human dignity and justice, tackling ageism and negative stereotypes about aging and sexuality, Jecker concludes that accessible sex robots for persons with disabilities are a reasonable way to support their sexuality.

A similar conclusion was reached by Fosch-Villaronga and Poulsen (2020), who argued that people with disabilities are frequently unable to enjoy physical touch, intimacy, and sexual pleasure in the same way as able-bodied people. They further point to the lack of support from health care services for the sexual needs of older adults, arguing for the sexual rights of older and disabled adults. This paper considers sex robots in comparison to 'sex care' defined as a…

> Sexual service for people with severe physical or mental disabilities (…) often done by professionals with a background in health care (…) focused on intimacy, physical touch and sexual satisfaction for disabled clients. (Nwanazia, 2018)

In Europe 12 organizations from seven countries—Belgium, Czech Republic, France, Italy, the Netherlands, Spain and Switzerland—form the European Platform Sexual Assistance for Persons with Disabilities (EPSEAS), delivering sex care to people with 'functional diversity' including physical disabilities. Fosch-Villaronga and Poulsen (2020) point out that sex care raises questions about the rights and status of sex workers and

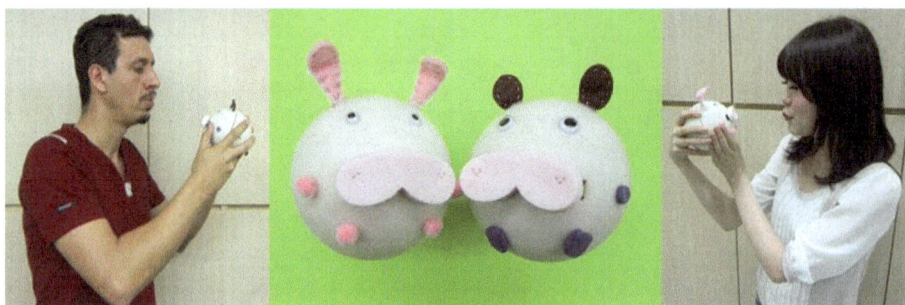

Image 8.4 Kissenger. *Credit* Hooman Samani (hoomansamani.com)

whether public funding can be used for these services. In addition to reviewing the features of existing sex robots, the authors also summarise the eight main legal and ethical implications of the use and development of robots for care purposes. These include human–robot safe interaction, allocation of responsibility and deception and infantilization (Fosch-Villaronga & Poulsen, 2020). The arguments for and against sex robots look set to continue.

8.5 Key Initiative—Lovotics[11]

Lovotics is a website with various research projects into human–robot relationships exploring love. Lovotics is run by a robotics researcher in the UK and currently offers several different types of Lovotics. The eponymous Lovotic is a tactile robot for an individual to interact with. Videos of its possible use can be found on the website. Kissenger is a robot to transfer kisses across distances. Using interactive digital media, Kissenger provides a physical interface for kissing when two people are apart. There are also potential Lovotics for human-to-robot kissing and human-to-virtual character kissing (Image 8.4).

8.6 Find Out More

- Importance of intimacy in later life: https://www.ncoa.org/article/why-is-intimacy-important-in-older-adults
- Examples of disability sex aids for couples and resources for people with different health conditions: https://www.intimaterider.com/

---

[11] http://www.lovotics.com/.

- Find out more about sex robots for aging and disability: https://www.vice.com/en/article/7k9bwq/sex-robots-should-target-the-elderly-and-the-disabled-experts-say.

References

Adams, M., Oye, J., & Parker, T. (2003). Sexuality of older adults and the Internet: From sex education to cybersex. *Sexual and Relationship Therapy, 18*(3), 405–415.

Angelini, L., Caon, M., Lalanne, D., Khaled, O.A. and Mugellini, E., (2014), September. Hugginess: Encouraging interpersonal touch through smart clothes. In Proceedings of the 2014 ACM International Symposium on Wearable Computers: Adjunct Program, 155-162.

Astell, A., & Clayton, D. (2024). "Like another human being in the room": A community case study of smart speakers to reduce loneliness in the oldest-old. *Frontier in Psychology, 15*, 1320555. https://doi.org/10.3389/fpsyg.2024.1320555

Bender, A. A., Burgess, E. O., & Barmon, C. (2020). Negotiating the lack of intimacy in assisted living: Resident desires, barriers, and strategies. *Journal of Applied Gerontology, 39*(1), 28–39.

Cha, J., Eid, M., Rahal, L., & Saddik, A. E. (2008). HugMe: An interpersonal haptic communication system. Haptic Audio Visual Environments and Games HAVE 2008. *IEEE International Workshop* (pp. 99–102). IEEE.

Cook, C., Schouten, V., Henrickson, M., & Mcdonald, S. (2017). Ethics, intimacy and sexuality in aged care. *Journal of Advanced Nursing, 73*, 3017–3027.

DiSalvo, C., Gemperle, F., Forlizzi, J., & Montgomery, E. (2003). The Hug: An exploration of robotic form for intimate communication. In *The 12th IEEE International Workshop on Robot and Human Interactive Communication, 2003. Proceedings* (pp. 403–408). ROMAN 2003. IEEE

Erens, B., Mitchell, K. R., Gibson, L., Datta, J., et al. (2019). Health status, sexual activity and satisfaction among older people in Britain: a mixed methods study. *PLoS One, 14*(3), e0213835. https://doi.org/10.1371/journal.pone.0213835

Fels, D. I., Smith, D. H., Baffa da Silva, R., Aybar, D., et al. (2015). IIS you is my digital baby: An intimate interface system for persons with disabilities. *GI '15: Proceedings of the 41st Graphics Interface Conference* (pp. 171–178).

Field, T. (2010). Touch for socioemotional and physical well-being: A review. *Developmental Review, 30*, 367–383.

Fosch-Villaronga, E., & Poulsen, A. (2020). Sex care robots: Exploring the potential use of sexual robot technologies for disabled and elder care. *Paladyn, Journal of Behavioral Robotics, 11*, 1–18.

Fromm-Reichmann, F. (1959). Loneliness. *Psychiatry, 22*(1), 1–15.

Garrett, D. (2014). Psychosocial barriers to sexual intimacy for older people. *British Journal of Nursing, 23*(6), 327–331.

Gersen, J. S. (2019). Sex Lex Machina. *Columbia Law Review, 119*(7), 1793–810.

Heatley Tejada, A., Dunbar, R., & Montero, M. (2020). Physical contact and loneliness: Being touched reduces perceptions of loneliness. *Adaptive Human Behavior and Physiology, 6*(3), 292–306.

Hinchliff, S., Tetley, J., Lee, D., & Nazroo, J. (2018). Older adults' experiences of sexual difficulties: Qualitative findings from the English Longitudinal Study on Ageing (ELSA). *The Journal of Sex Research, 55*(2), 152–163.

Jecker, N. S. (2021). Nothing to be ashamed of: Sex robots for older adults with disabilities. *Journal of Medical Ethics, 47*, 26–32.

Karam, M., Branje, C., Price, E., Russo, F., et al. (2008). Towards a model human cochlea: Sensory substitution for crossmodal audio-tactile displays. *Proceedings of Graphics Interface 2008* (pp. 267–274). Windsor.

Lomanowska, A. M., & Guitton, M. J. (2016). Online intimacy and well-being in the digital age. *Internet Interventions, 4*(2), 138–144.

Macleod, A. (2020). *The Over 45s Adult Sexuality and Intimacy Scale: A new approach to understanding and measuring sexuality in mid and later life.* Doctoral Thesis submitted to Swinburne University of Technology, Australia.

Malta. (2007). Love Actually! Older adults and their romantic internet relationships. *Australian Journal of Emerging Technologies and Society, 5*(2), 84–102.

Minarcik, J., Wetterneck, C. T., & Short, M. B. (2016). The effects of sexually explicit material use on romantic relationship dynamics. *Journal of Behavioral Addictions, 5*(4), 700–707. https://doi.org/10.1556/2006.5.2016.078

Motamedi, N. (2007). Keep in touch: a tactile-vision intimate interface. In *TEI '07: Proceedings of the 1st International Conference on Tangible and Embedded Interaction* (pp. 21–22).

Mulleler, F., Vetere, F., Gibbs, M. R., Kjeldskov, J., et al. (2005). Hug over a distance. *CHI EA '05: CHI '05 Extended Abstracts on Human Factors in Computing Systems* (pp. 1673–1676).

Nwanazia, C. (2018). Sex Care in The Netherlands—Helping the Disabled Find Intimacy, *Dutch Review.* Available at: https://dutchreview.com/culture/love-dating/sex-care-in-the-Netherlands-helping-the-disabled-find-intimacy/

Scandurra, C., Mezza, F., Esposito, C., Vitelli, R., et al. (2022). Online sexual activities in Italian older adults: The role of gender, sexual orientation, and permissiveness. *Sexuality Research and Social Policy, 19,* 248–263. https://doi.org/10.1007/s13178-021-00538-1

Simpson, P., Horne, M., Browne, J., Brown Wilson, C., et al. (2017). Old(er) care home residents and sexual/intimate citizenship. *Ageing and Society, 37,* 243–265.

Sternberg, R. J. (1986). A triangular theory of love. *Psychological Review, 93*(2), 119–135. https://doi.org/10.1037/0033-295X.93.2.119

Sullivan, H. S. (1955). *The Interpersonal Theory of Psychiatry.* Routledge.

Teh, J. K. S., Cheok, A. D., Peiris, R. L., Choi, Y., et al. (2008). Huggy Pajama: A mobile parent and child hugging communication system. In *Proceedings of the 7th International Conference on Interaction Design and Children* (pp. 250–257). ACM.

Tsetserukou, D. (2010). HaptiHug: A novel haptic display for communication of hug over a distance. In A. M. L. Kappers, J. B. F. van Erp, W. M. Bergmann Tiest & F. C. T. van der Helm (Eds.), *Haptics: Generating and Perceiving Tangible Sensations. EuroHaptics 2010. Lecture Notes in Computer Science* (Vol. 6191). Springer. https://doi.org/10.1007/978-3-642-14064-8_49

Weiss, R. S. (1973). *Loneliness: The Experience of Emotional and Social Isolation.* The MIT Press.

Zeedyk, S. (2006). From subjectivity to intersubjectivity: The transformative roles of emotional intimacy and imitation. *Infant and Child Development, 15,* 321–344.

Staying Connected to Healthcare 9

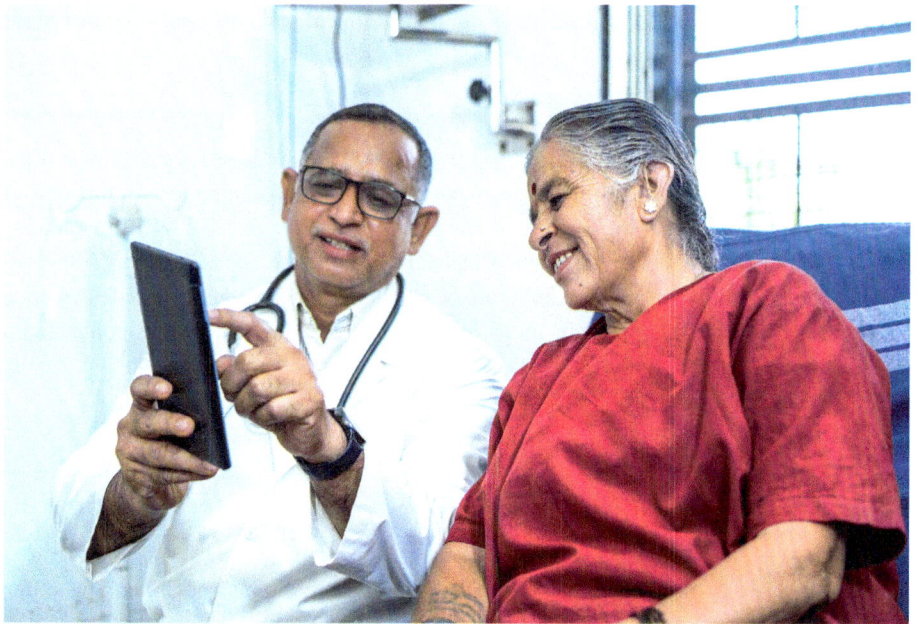

Image 9.1 *Credit* Shutterstock–Westock productions

9.1 The Challenge

Age increases the risk for many health conditions including cardiovascular disease, cancer, type 2 diabetes, and dementia (Image 9.1). Various factors contribute to increased risk of developing age-related conditions including general wear and tear on our body, exposure to environmental pollutants, and lifestyle factors such as diet, alcohol consumption, smoking, and physical activity. Health problems are found to amplify the problems of loneliness for older adults by reducing social contact. As has been indicated, the experiences of mental illness, for example, have been found to have an impact on loneliness by limiting social interaction.

Some of these factors may be modifiable and individual risk is also moderated by hereditary factors. However, many people find themselves managing one or more medical conditions, which requires frequent interactions with healthcare services and professionals. Staying connected to healthcare is, therefore, a vital part of active aging and covers all aspects of care from assessments, consultations, clinical sessions, and support groups.

9.2 What's in This Chapter?

Given the prevalence of health conditions in later life, this has been the area of most development in respect of technology. These are largely the preserve of AGE-WELL Challenge Area 2: Health Care and Health Service Delivery, with those focused on reducing risk and promoting healthy behaviours and part of Challenge Area 6: Healthy Lifestyles and Wellness. As such this chapter will focus on AgeTech keeping older adults connected to healthcare services, professionals, support, and information, specifically apps, telehealth, online resources and chatbots.

9.3 Persona and Scenario: Mei[1]

Persona: Mei is a 71-year-old Buddhist woman who lives in Shanghai, China. She suffers from coronary heart disease, dizziness, and vascular headaches, and is taking 'quick-acting' heart pills, Betalloc tablets and Saridon. She also had a mastectomy for breast cancer more than ten years ago. At present, her husband lives in a government-run nursing home, costing more than 3000 yuan a month. Mei is alone at home with a pet dog. Her family has a good economic situation. Her pension is more than 4000 yuan (US $619) each month, while her husband's pension is more than 6000 yuan (US $929). Both her son and daughter-in-law are doctors. Mei's living environment is good, with elevators,

---

[1] Case study created by Dr. Fang Yang. Associate Professor, Department of Social Work, School of Sociology and Political Science, Shanghai University.

parking lots and other necessary living facilities. When she sees a doctor who prescribes her medicine, she drives her car to the nearest community health service centre.

Mei goes to the nursing home to take care of her husband. Sometimes she also goes to her brother's home to visit her aged mother. Also, she has to pick up her grandson from the kindergarten, do housework and feed stray cats.

Scenario: Mei worries that if she is sick or has a heart attack, no one will call an ambulance or accompany her to the hospital. The risk of living alone is too high. However, technology helps her manage her loneliness. She loves cats and dogs, so if anything interesting happens, she will take a video and post it to her WeChat group, and then her friends in the group will see the news she shares. Or if she wants to organize a gathering, she will invite her friends in the WeChat group, just saying "Get together!", then her friends will come to her home for dinner. She usually makes coffee for them, and they have a chat. When she wants to eat, she can use her mobile phone to order takeout, which is very convenient. Mei hopes the community can provide more home services such as home massages and housework but she thinks the services should be paid for by the government. Now she is ready to sell her house and move into her son's neighbourhood.

Mei can be considered fairly typical of many older people who are living with chronic conditions. However, she is currently independent and still driving and compared to lots of older people, is in a secure financial position. Mei is also a proactive technology user, contacting her friends and sharing information, particularly via WeChat, China's major social media platform. Although she remains active and has friends who can visit or chat with, Mei is concerned that in a crisis no one would be there for her. She could benefit from a system to help her self-manage her coronary heart disease and connect with her clinical support team to keep track of adverse events. She could also discuss sharing updates with her family so that they are alerted if a problem occurs.

9.4 Technology for Connecting to Healthcare

9.4.1 Self-management Tools

Given the prevalence of heart disease in later life, a range of self-management apps are available in many countries. Typically, these include an app for patients to manage their condition, including symptoms, daily routine, and medication. Additionally, there may be a web portal providing direct links to the clinical team. In China, where chronic heart disease is the second leading cause of death, WeChat, which Mei already uses, is becoming a common platform for self-management. WeChat, which has more than one billion users, has been proposed as a tool for the self-management of chronic diseases including chronic heart disease (Chen et al., 2020). Researchers have found that interventions using WeChat can improve adherence to cardio-protective medication regimes (Ni et al., 2018), and support cardiac rehabilitation and secondary prevention with high acceptance from users (Dorje et al., 2018).

In late 2019, AI Nurse[2] was launched on WeChat as a platform for patients to manage their heart disease from home by connecting them with nurses in the community. Developed as a collaboration between Novartis and Tencent, the impact on patient health and other outcomes is currently being investigated. Between July 2020 and January 2021, more than 25,000 patients were recruited from 300+ China's leading hospitals across 100 cities to use AI nurses to manage their chronic heart disease.

For Canadians living with chronic heart disease, 'Medly',[3] an innovation from the University Health Network in Toronto, comprises an app and clinician dashboard to support self-management. Similarly, the 'MyHeart'[4] app is available for UK patients to self-manage their daily lives and allow their clinical team to receive notifications, messages and important notices. The online MyHeart platform also includes educational videos to support people with their rehabilitation and medication monitoring. Other heart health self-management tools are currently being tested around the world including HappyHeart (Heiney et al., 2020) in the USA, HeartCare+ in the Middle East (Elsayad et al., 2017) and Care4MyHeart, co-created with patients and other stakeholders in Australia (Woods et al., 2019).

P-STEP®[5] is a new app funded by the European Space Agency, co-designed by clinicians, researchers at the University of Leicester and patients living with long-term conditions. P-STEP® is intended to support and promote exercise—specifically walking—for people with long-term conditions. Currently, P-STEP® is supporting heart diseases, lung diseases and Type 2 Diabetes Mellitus. Along with walking advice, P-STEP® provides information on air quality and pollen to allow a user to pick the best walk at the best time to avoid pollution. Future developments requested by users include sharing favourite walks and socially connecting to compare their progress. Although designed for people with long-term conditions, P-STEP® can be used by anyone who wishes to walk in better-quality air (Image 9.2).

9.4.2 Telehealth/Telemedicine

Telehealth refers to healthcare services delivered to patients by providers who are in another location. Telehealth can be delivered to a patient's home or using specific video-conferencing facilities in community clinics. One of the largest telehealth networks is the

---

[2] https://www.novartis.com/stories/patient-perspectives/ai-nurse-evolving-health-failure-patients-china.

[3] https://medly.ca/.

[4] https://mymhealth.com/myheart.

[5] https://business.esa.int/projects/p-step.

9.4 Technology for Connecting to Healthcare

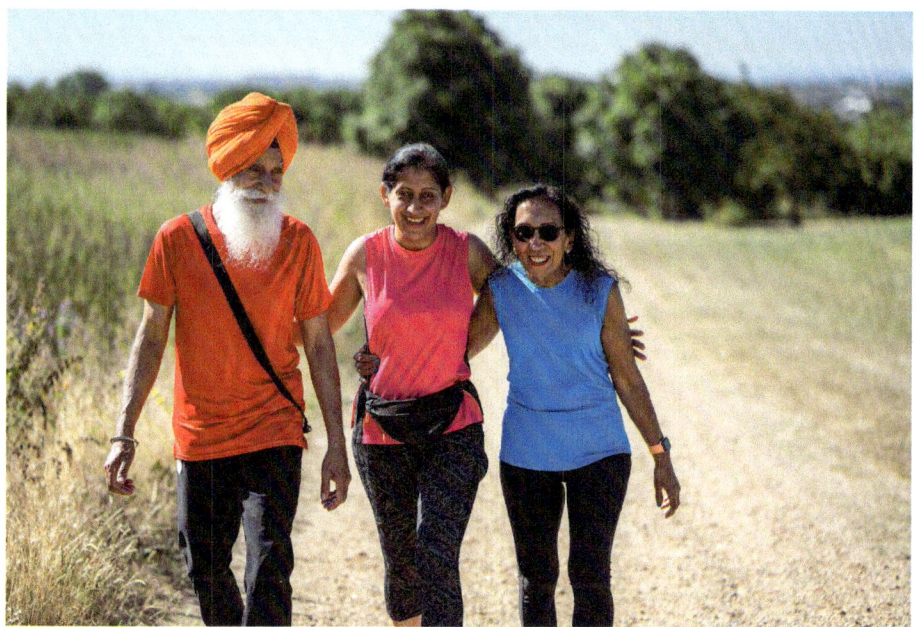

Image 9.2 *Credit* Peter Kindersley/ageing better

Ontario Telemedicine Network in Canada[6] which includes all public hospitals, clinics, family health teams, physician offices, nursing stations, medical and nursing schools, professional organizations, Community Care Access Centres, First Nations Communities, long-term care homes, educational facilities and public health. OTN serves as the platform for delivering remote care and in 2020 delivered more than one million virtual visits. Telehealth has been hailed as a major breakthrough in healthcare. According to the WHO telehealth…

> Can contribute to achieving universal health coverage by improving access for patients to quality, cost-effective, health services wherever they may be. It is particularly valuable for those in remote areas, vulnerable groups and aging populations. (WHO, 2016)

9.4.3 Online Resources

Web-based support groups and online communities are well-established resources for people to stay connected to healthcare (Image 9.3). Support groups and communities provide the opportunity to interact with others in the same situation, share experiences and ask questions in a safe environment. Such interactions provide reassurance to individuals that

---

[6] https://otn.ca/.

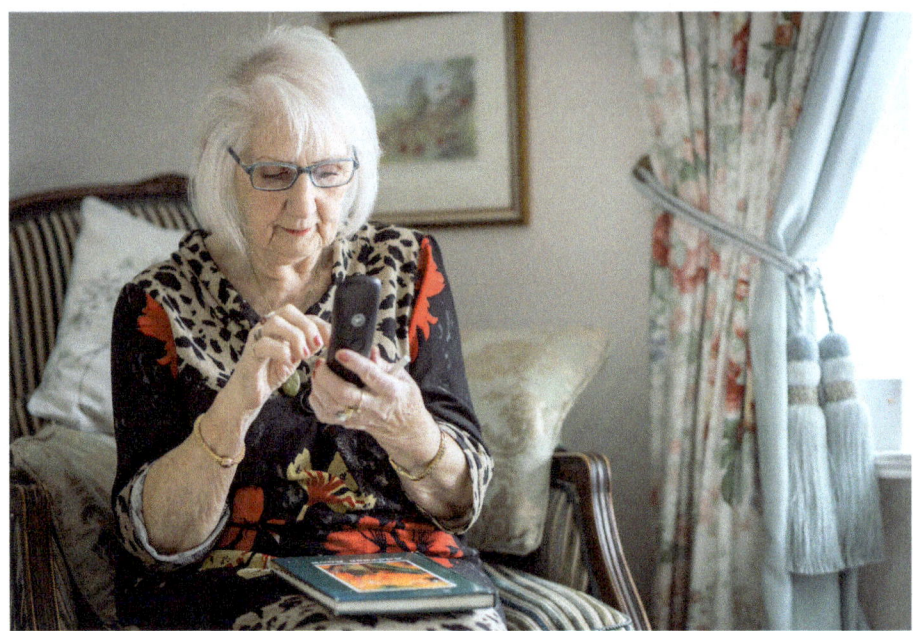

Image 9.3 *Credit* Independent age/ageing better

they are not going through this situation alone and to receive emotional support (Solberg, 2014). Online communities are also a source of information about health conditions, symptom management and treatments (Solberg, 2014).

One popular site is 'PatientsLikeMe' (PLM), an online platform for people living with any health condition to connect with other people living with the same condition to share their experiences and 'take control of their health'.[7] Established initially to bring together individuals living with Amyotrophic Lateral Sclerosis (ALS), it expanded in 2011 for people with any condition to come together. Currently, users of PLM are tracking more than 2800 health conditions, sharing experiences and tips on nutrition, sleep, and relaxation. Another key feature of PLM, which makes it an interesting example of the potential of online communities, is the research it carries out. This includes analysis of the data reported by the approximately 830,000 users and also patient-initiated projects, both of which are analyzed and reported in various peer-reviewed publications (e.g., Wicks et al., 2019; Wild et al., 2018).[8] Examination of PLM users' motivation to participate in patient-led research includes…

---

[7] https://www.patientslikeme.com/.

[8] Full set of PLM patient-led research can be found here: https://patientslikeme-bibliography.s3.amazonaws.com/PLM%20Research%20Manuscripts%20Bibliography.pdf.

9.4 Technology for Connecting to Healthcare

> ... facilitating provider-patient communication, improving comprehension of medical information, understanding their disease, and bringing a more individualized approach to health care. (Bradley et al., 2016, p. 2)

These findings are relevant for the greater inclusion of patients in research design and decision-making across all health conditions, especially older or disabled patients who are often excluded from these processes (Astell & Fels, 2021).

In addition to this multi-condition platform, there are also many condition-specific support groups and online communities for most late-life common conditions. These are often managed by national organizations. For example, people living with cancer in Canada can go to 'CancerConnection.ca' to *'share their experiences and build supportive relationships'*.[9] For people living with Parkinson's disease, the Michael J. Fox Foundation hosts the 'Parkinson's Buddy Network', an online community to help people make 'meaningful connections'.[10] For those in the UK, the NHS Apps library includes 'HealthUnlocked', a service where people can connect to more than 700 online communities for a wide range of conditions.[11]

In addition to online communities, online educational resources can also help keep people connected through interacting with professionals who deliver courses or respond to queries posted on the site. For example, Parkinson Canada hosts webinars for people to find out more about living with Parkinson's disease,[12] while those with cardiovascular problems can view webinars from Heart and Stroke.[13] People wanting to find out more about age-related memory changes can access the Baycrest Health Sciences online Memory and Aging Program,[14] developed to extend the long-established in-person version to people anywhere (Yusopov et al., 2022).

People can also connect with others at online activities such as the DATE Lab/AcToDementia bi-weekly sessions introducing tablet games for dementia[15] or join a Massive Open Online Course (MOOC) such as the one about managing Type 2 Diabetes offered by hospitals in Scotland (Mackenzie et al., 2021). MOOCs are free, open courses accessible to anyone usually offered by universities and other institutions. While MOOCs typically have limited direct interaction with tutors, they do offer opportunities to connect with others studying the course.

---

[9] https://action.cancer.ca/en/living-with-cancer/how-we-can-help/connect-with-our-online-community.
[10] https://parkinsonsbuddynetwork.michaeljfox.org/.
[11] https://healthunlocked.com/.
[12] https://www.parkinson.ca/resources/webinars/.
[13] https://www.heartandstroke.ca/what-we-do/webinars.
[14] https://shop.baycrest.org/products/memory-and-aging-online-program.
[15] https://www.date-lab.com/programs.

Educational resources are also available for people who find themselves providing care for a family member. This can be particularly important for families caring for relatives with neurodegenerative conditions, such as Alzheimer's disease and other forms of dementia, which can place significant demands on caregivers. Online education for family caregivers, which has been demonstrated to be equivalent to in-person, has the added benefit of remote and asynchronous delivery, both of which increase accessibility (Scerbe et al., 2023). This is particularly important for families living in rural or remote areas who experience long wait lists for specialist services, often accompanied by limited resources, information and education (Kosteniuk et al., 2016). Available resources include Caregiving Strategies,[16] and the Family Caregiver Alliance,[17] both of which target the needs of family caregivers.

9.4.4 Chatbots

Chatbots or conversational agents have become familiar to many people through voice-activated systems such as 'Alexa' (Amazon) and 'Siri' (Apple). These computer programs are scripted to respond to common questions and queries and can interact with humans through speech or text. The use of chatbots in healthcare is on the rise as a means of supporting people to live with many health conditions, by providing direct interaction, immediate response and reducing demands on healthcare staff. Multiple benefits of chatbots on mobile devices have been proposed including users not needing to download or learn to use a new app as the chatbot can work within existing messaging platforms (e.g., WhatsApp; CAH, 2018).

A one-year evaluation of Vik, a chatbot developed in France for patients with breast cancer, found that the more often people interacted with Vik, the better their medication adherence (Chaix et al., 2019). Another group in France developed a chatbot specifically for older people receiving chemotherapy at home to conduct monitoring evaluations and free up nurses (Piau et al., 2019). For people living with chronic heart disease, 'Roborto', a chatbot developed in Italy is intended to encourage medication adherence through text-based natural conversation and update the clinical team on progress (Fadhil, 2018). An example of a voice-based conversational agent is 'Lena', developed by a team in Switzerland specifically for older adults living with chronic obstructive pulmonary disease (Cleres et al., 2021). Presented as a 'digital member of the medical team', 'Lena' provides remote monitoring of symptoms, which users felt they could use daily as part of their self-management routine. Such developments with voice technology could also be useful for people living with dementia, for whom the potential of chatbots is currently underdeveloped (Ruggiano et al., 2021).

---

[16] https://rgps.on.ca/about-the-online-course/.
[17] https://www.caregiver.org/resource/fca-webinars/.

9.5 Key Initiative—Keeping Indigenous Older People Connected to Healthcare

In this section, we consider projects exploring the role of technology in keeping indigenous older adults connected to healthcare. A review by Canadian researchers identified a lack of technology developed with and for older Indigenous communities (Jones et al., 2017). In response, the Aging Technologies for Indigenous Communities in Ontario (ATI-CON) project set out to examine the current use of technology by older rural/remote and Indigenous populations across regions of Saskatchewan and Ontario.[18] Key outputs included a guidebook and infographic (Image 9.4) for organizations seeking to partner with indigenous communities in technology assessment and development. Current research is examining the potential of wearable technologies to allow indigenous communities, including those living with dementia, to age in place (Jacklin et al., 2020) while research at the University of Saskatchewan is exploring how telehealth services can support older Indigenous people in leading a healthy lifestyle.

Work with Australian Aboriginal communities has identified the importance of social interaction in a model of healthy aging, which includes culturally safe care, that could be delivered through technology (Wettasinghe et al., 2020). In respect of staying connected to healthcare, the Australian Integrated Mental Health Initiative (AIMHI) was established to produce resources for dealing with mental health problems in remote communities. One output, the AIMHI Stay Strong App, was developed to promote well-being and improve connections between Indigenous communities and service providers.[19]

9.6 Find Out More

- Personalised integrated care in the UK: http://www.ageuk.org.uk/our-impact/programmes/integrated-care/
- National Digital Healthcare Mission launched in India to develop integrated digital health infrastructure to benefit older people: https://unravel.ink/helping-indias-elderly-cross-the-digital-divide-as-the-country-ages/
- How digital healthcare in Latin America can enhance efficacy and improve delivery: https://cacm.acm.org/magazines/2020/11/248215-digital-healthcare-in-latin-america/fulltext.

---

[18] https://www.i-caare.ca/technology-for-aging.
[19] https://www.menzies.edu.au/page/Research/Projects/Mental_Health_and_wellbeing/Development_of_the_Stay_Strong_iPad_App/.

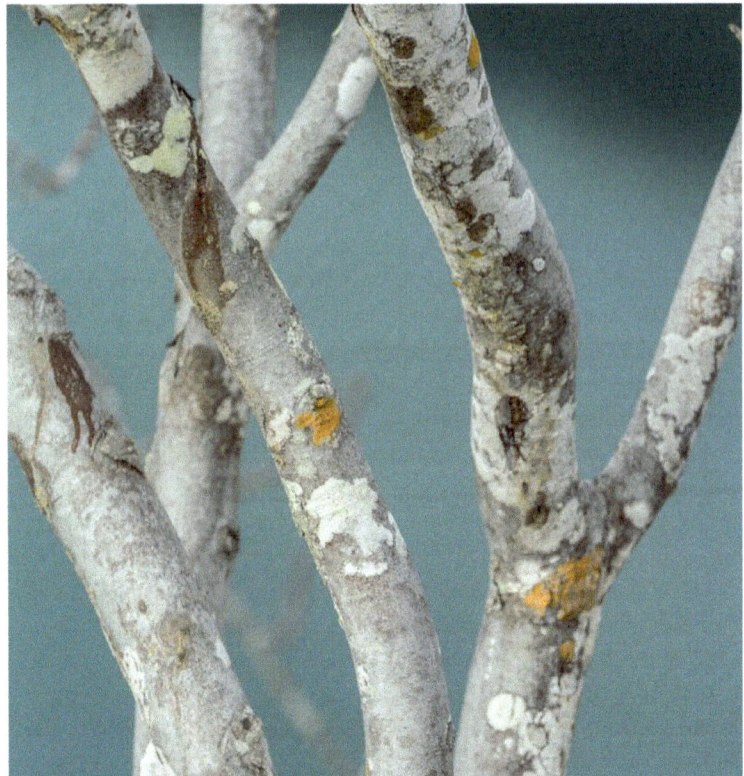

Image 9.4 ATICON infographic. *Credit* Aging Technologies for Indigenous Communities in Ontario (ATICON) infographic—a guide for partnering with Indigenous communities and organizations to conduct technology development research

References

Astell, A. J., & Fels, D. I. (2021). Co-production methods in health research. In A. Sixsmith, J. Sixsmith, A. Mihailidis & M. L. Fang (Eds.), *Knowledge, Innovation and Impact in Health—A Handbook for the Engaged Researcher* (pp. 175–182). Springer.

References

Bradley, M., Braverman, J., Harrington, M., & Wicks, P. (2016). Patients' motivations and interest in research: characteristics of volunteers for patient-led projects on PatientsLikeMe. *BMC Research Involvement and Engagement, 2*(33). https://doi.org/10.1186/s40900-016-0047-6

Centre for Advanced Hindsight. Chatbots for diabetes self-management. (2018). Available at https://advanced-hindsight.com/wp-content/uploads/2018/02/Chatbots-for-Diabetes-Self-Management.pdf

Chaix, B., Bibault, J. E., Pienkowski, A., Delamon, G., et al. (2019). When chatbots meet patients: One-year prospective study of conversations between patients with breast cancer and a chatbot. *Journal of Medial Internet Research Cancer, 5*(1), e12856. https://doi.org/10.2196/12856

Chen, X., Zhou, X., Li, H., Li, J., et al. (2020). The value of WeChat application in chronic disease management in China. *Computer Methods and Programmes in Biomedicine, 196*, 105710. https://doi.org/10.1016/j.cmpb.2020.105710

Cleres, D., Rassouli, F., Brutsche, M., & Kowatsch, T. (2021). Lena: A voice-based conversational agent for remote patient monitoring in chronic obstructive pulmonary disease. In *Joint Proceedings of the ACM IUI 2021 Workshops*, April 13–17, 2021, College Station, USA.

Dorje, T., Zhao, G., Scheer, A., Tsokey, L. et al.(2018). SMARTphone and social media-based cardiac rehabilitation and secondary prevention (SMART-CRISP) for patients with coronary heart disease in China: A randomised controlled trial protocol, *BMJ Open, 8*(6). e021908. https://doi.org/10.1136/bmjopen-2018-021908

Elsayed, H. A. G., Galal, M. A., & Syed, L. (2017). HeartCare+: A smart heart care mobile application for Framingham-based early risk prediction of hard coronary heart diseases in Middle East. *Mobile Information Systems, 1*, 1–11. https://doi.org/10.1155/2017/9369532

Fadhil, A. (2018). A conversational interface to improve medication adherence: Towards AI Support in patient's treatment. arXiv:1803.09844. https://doi.org/10.48550/arXiv.1803.09844

Heiney, S. P., Donevant, S. B., Arp Adams, S., Parker, P. D., et al. (2020). A smartphone app for self-management of heart failure in older African Americans: Feasibility and usability study. *Journal of Medical Internet Research Aging, 3*(1), e17142. https://doi.org/10.2196/17142

Jacklin, K., Pitawanakwat, K., Blind, M., Lemieux, A. M. et al. (2020). Peace of mind: A community-industry-academic partnership to adapt dementia technology for Anishinaabe communities on Manitoulin Island. *Journal of Rehabilitation and Assistive Technologies Engineering, 16*(7), 1–11. https://doi.org/10.1177/2055668320958327

Jones, L., Jacklin, K., & O'Connell, M. E. (2017). Development and use of health-related technologies in indigenous communities: Critical review. *Journal of Medical Internet Research, 19*(7), e256. https://doi.org/10.2196/jmir.7520

Kosteniuk, J., Morgan, D., O'Connell, M. E., Dal Bello-Haas, V., et al. (2016). Focus on dementia care: Continuing education preferences, challenges, and catalysts among rural home care providers. *Educational Gerontology, 42*, 608–620. https://doi.org/10.1080/03601277.2016.1205404

Mackenzie, S. C., Cumming, K. M., Garrell, D., Brodie, D., et al. (2021). Massive open online course for type 2 diabetes self-management: Adapting education in the COVID-19 era. *BMJ Innovations, 7*(1), 141–147. https://doi.org/10.1136/bmjinnov-2020-000526

Ni, Z., Liu, C., Wu, B., Yang, Q., et al. (2018). A mHealth intervention to improve medication adherence among patients with coronary heart disease in China: Development of an intervention. *International Journal of Nursing Science, 5*(4), 322–330.

Piau, A., Crissey, R., Brechemier, D., Balardy, L., et al. (2019). A smartphone chatbot application to optimize monitoring of older patients with cancer. *International Journal of Medical Informatics, 128*(14), 18–25. https://doi.org/10.1016/j.ijmedinf.2019.05.013

Ruggiano, N., Brown, E. L., Roberts, L., Framil Suarez, C. V., et al. (2021). Chatbots to support people with dementia and their caregivers: Systematic review of functions and quality. *Journal of Medical Internet Research, 23*(6). e25006. https://doi.org/10.2196/25006

Scerbe, A., O'Connell, M. E., Astell, A., Morgan, D., et al. (2023). Digital tools for delivery of dementia education for caregivers of persons with dementia: A systematic review and meta-analysis. *PLoS ONE, 18*(5), e0283600. https://doi.org/10.1371/journal.pone.0283600

Solberg, L. (2014). The benefits of online health communities. *Virtual Mentor, 16*(4), 270–274. https://doi.org/10.1001/virtualmentor.2014.16.4.stas1-1404

Wettasinghe, P. M., Allan, W., Garvey, G., Timbery, A., et al. (2020). Older Aboriginal Australians' health concerns and preferences for healthy ageing programs. *International Journal of Environmental Research and Public Health, 17*(20), 7390. https://doi.org/10.3390/ijerph17207390

World Health Organisation (WHO). (2016). Global Diffusion of eHealth: Making Universal Health Coverage Achievable. Report of the third global survey on eHealth. Available at: https://www.who.int/publications/i/item/9789241511780

Wicks, P., McCaffrey, S., Goodwin, K., Black, R., et al. (2019). A modular Health-Related Quality of Life Instrument for electronic assessment and treatment monitoring: Web-based development and psychometric validation of core thrive items. *Journal of Medical Internet Research, 21*(1), e12075. https://doi.org/10.2196/12075

Wild, M. G., Ostini, R., Harrington, M., Cavanaugh, K. L., et al. (2018). Validation of the shortened perceived medical condition self-management scale in patients with chronic disease. *Psychological Assessment, 30*(10), 1300–1307.

Woods, L., Duff., J., Roehrer, E., Walker, K., et al. (2019). Design of a consumer mobile health app for heart failure: Findings from the nurse-led co-design of Care4myHeart. *Journal of Medical Internet Research Nursing, 2*(1), e14633. https://doi.org/10.2196/14633

Yusopov, I., VanderMorris, S., Rich, J., Astell, A. J., et al. (2022). An agile development cycle of an online memory program for healthy older adults. *Canadian Journal on Aging/La Revue Canadienne Du Vieillissement, 41*(4), 647–656.

Staying Connected and the Digital Divide 10

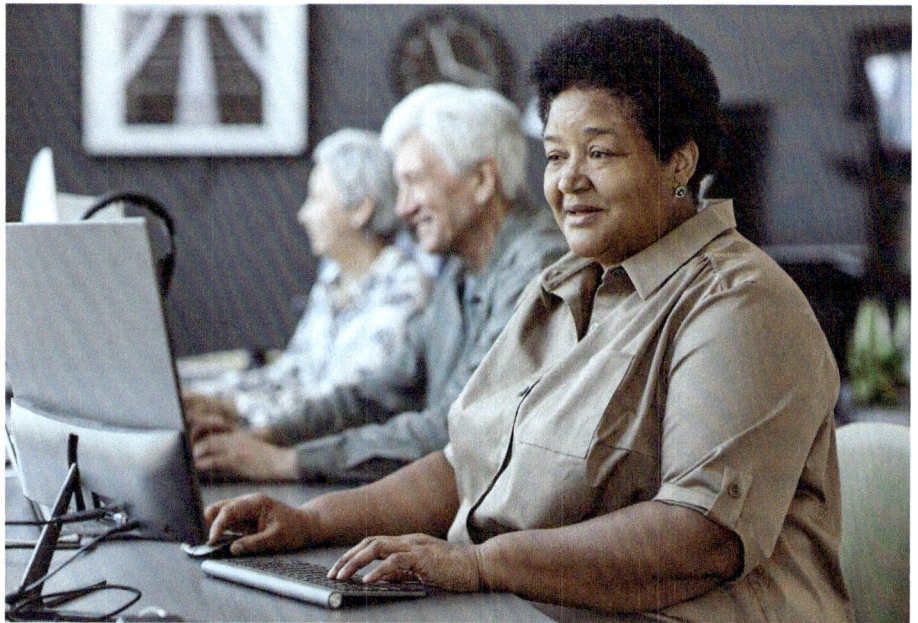

Image 10.1 *Credit* Shutterstock—SeventyFour

10.1 The Challenge

The focus of this book on AgeTech for staying connected has highlighted two things: (1) how important staying connected is for human beings; and (2) the range of technology available to assist people to stay connected as they age. While these technologies offer opportunities for people to stay connected, it is important to address the many barriers to access and use that prevent getting these technologies into people's hands (Image 10.1). An important challenge for policymakers and service providers in the post-pandemic world is the 'digital divide'. Exploring the digital divide could be a book in its own right and draws upon sociological as well as psychological and behavioural factors. The term digital divide is used to describe patterns of unequal access to digital technologies based on demographic factors like age, disability, gender, ethnicity, income, and education, (Mossberger et al., 2003). Although the COVID-19 pandemic did find older adults developing new skills and confidence in using digital technologies, it also presented new challenges for those who did not.

10.2 What's in This Chapter?

This chapter explores the issue of the digital divide and the need to address this in policy. The story of Roxanne and her husband Mike sets the scene. There are differences in the use of AgeTech based on poor access to infrastructure like broadband, poor access to devices and equipment like computers, and a lack of skills, motivation, and support for older adults to use digital technologies. The pandemic highlighted the digital divide further with the increased need to use technology such as the Internet to access services, attend medical appointments, stay in touch with family, and friends and do online shopping.

10.3 Persona and Scenario: Roxanne[1]

Persona: Mike and Roxanne live on a farm in a rural area of Canada. Roxanne sits on the corner of the bed she shares with Mike, while he is resting on the couch, giving her a few minutes to catch up on email. She is wary about leaving him unattended because lately, he has been having particularly confused days. They live too remotely to receive any formal homecare services provided by the health region. They were briefly able to hire someone privately with the support of the individualised funding program offered by the health region. To receive this funding, they had to acknowledge they could not also use formal

---

[1] Case study created by Dr. Megan O'Connell, Clinical Psychologist, Rural and Remote Memory Services Saskatchewan and University of Saskatchewan.

10.3 Persona and Scenario: Roxanne

homecare or day programming. Unfortunately, this hired worker was unable to manage when Mike's symptoms of dementia became more pronounced. Roxanne currently has active adverts looking for a replacement caregiver but recruitment in this isolated farming region is challenging. Her caregiving duties are currently 24/7, and she finds herself thankful for Mike's loud snoring because she can confirm he is sleeping in the next room.

Scenario: The only Internet access is via cell tower, and she can only get reliable cellular data access in this one spot in her house when she sits on the leftmost corner of the bed. Otherwise, accessing the weak cell signal requires Roxanne to walk up the ridge in the backyard. On this occasion, she can connect and check her email but there has been no response to her adverts. One email is a reminder of the Telehealth video-conferenced support group for spousal caregivers of persons with dementia that she tries to attend every month. She has been attending this group for several years with caregivers from across the province who are also caring for a spouse with atypical young-onset dementia. She would love to attend this support group meeting, which she sees as her personal sanctuary. She knows, however, that she cannot attend this month's support group. No one is available to look after Mike. Also, she is on her last tank of gas and is not sure if she can afford to travel the 40 km to the nearest small town where she can access the health region's Telehealth suite. Here she could use the equipment and secure broadband access for seamless videoconferencing.

Although the Provincial Telehealth Network has opened up in recent months for joining desktop solutions with the videoconferencing provided in the Telehealth suites, her cellular data would not support videoconferencing. The only other option for broadband access on the farm is satellite service, which is way too costly each month. Monthly expenses take up as much of her mental energy as cleaning up after Mike's frequent occurrences of incontinence. Roxanne had to give up her work when caregiving for Mike became too stressful. First, she took a stress leave, which then turned into a longer-term leave, and the disability income was not enough. Mike has been unable to work since the age of 52, not long after his diagnosis of dementia due to frontotemporal dementia. Their hobby farm became too much for Roxanne to manage on her own and they have sold most of the revenue generating animals. Since then, they have struggled to get by from month to month. She types out a message for the support group with the keyboard on her cell phone—hoping this attempt at an asynchronous form of connection will help her feel less helpless and alone.

Solution: Roxanne's situation is sadly not uncommon among people who become caregivers for family members. Given the progressive nature of dementia, Roxanne, like many family caregivers, has gradually found herself providing more and more care for Mike. This has led to her becoming disconnected from her community and potential support mechanisms, which is compounded by living in a remote area. She currently does not have any respite from caregiving and is unable to access the caregiving support that is available remotely. Living in a remote area, they are among the thousands who struggle to

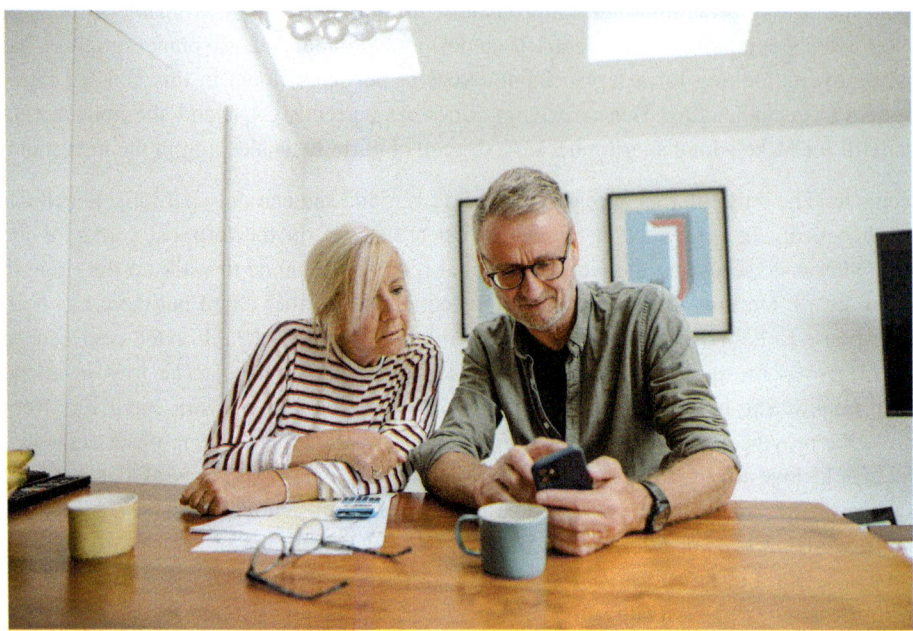

Image 10.2 Independent age/ageing better

access vital contact and services. Roxanne desperately needs to be connected to support for her and Mike but is unable to access them. In their case, remoteness is one problem that is often compounded by financial challenges.

The first step to helping Roxanne and Mike is to provide reliable Internet access. Arguably, Roxanne is providing a vital service by caring for Mike full-time. Providing them with a satellite service that ensures Internet connectivity could radically alter their situation, at a fraction of the cost of long-term care. Reliable Internet would give them both access to remote consultations with their family health team, memory services and Alzheimer's Society. Roxanne could access Internet resources for caregivers and deal with banking and other essential services remotely. While she is without a second caregiver, Roxanne has to manage with asynchronous support, but reliable Internet access could give her immediate access to other caregivers, for example through a blue-tooth headset she could wear even when she is with Mike (Image 10.2).

10.4 Understanding Digital Exclusion and the Digital Divide

The case of Roxanne and Mike illustrates the importance of addressing digital exclusion in older age. Later life comes with barriers and challenges to pursuing social connections. Mobility may decline, and we may become unable to drive or have limited access to

10.4 Understanding Digital Exclusion and the Digital Divide

public transport to see people in person. Older adults increasingly need access to communication technologies. Those who do not have access will have problems participating in social life, for example, communicating with other people or accessing services such as healthcare, that require the use of these technologies. The increased use of digital technologies to support aging can be seen as a double-edged sword. On the one side, internet-enabled resources have the potential to enhance life by creating new social networks and opportunities. On the other side, increased use of online tools can consolidate existing disadvantages and create new inequalities. As we become increasingly entangled with digital tools, exclusion from it becomes a new form of inequality. A first step towards understanding the issue is therefore to recognise these inequalities.

The local disparities or gaps between individuals and households using technologies in different countries need to be understood through the cultural, social, political, and economic conditions which inform everyday experiences (Tsatsou, 2011). There may be a range of individual, social, economic, and cultural challenges that see older adults in different locations excluded from or accessing technologies. However, the digital divide between those who have access to technology and those who do not is a global issue with similar challenges existing for older adults regardless of borders. Getting access to infrastructure and equipment and developing the skills to use digital technologies are common issues. In China, for example, during the pandemic, there was an increase in using technologies like smartphones for virus tracking which meant that older people were often reliant on other people like family for technological support, with those on low incomes and living in rural areas without access to the internet potentially digitally excluded (Yao et al., 2021). These issues were also found in the person and scenario of Roxanne and Mark in Canada.

A correlation between age, digital exclusion, and disadvantage has been found to exist (Damant & Knapp, 2015). In January 2021, approximately 22 million older Americans, equating to 42% of the over 65 s, lacked broadband access at home, according to a report released by the Older Adults Technology Services, Inc. (OATS), and the Humana Foundation. The implications include a lack of access to social services, digital healthcare (including Telehealth and apps for managing chronic conditions), public health information, and the increased risk of social isolation (OATS, 2021). As with any other form of technology, those in need of Telehealth must have access to the Internet and also any devices required to interact with the healthcare provider. Having to travel to the nearest clinic with video-conferencing facilities is not practical for large numbers of people. This digital divide, therefore, presents an urgent social and health crisis not just in the United States, but across the world.

10.4.1 Getting Access to the Internet When on Low Income

A primary issue of the digital divide is affordable access to the Internet. Even in wealthier countries like the UK, it is estimated 100,000 households in the UK did not have access to the Internet due to costs with a further two million households having difficulties affording this (Ofcom, 2022). Many older adults across the world live on fixed incomes which put Internet access out of reach. OECD data for 2018 identified levels of Pensioner Poverty in selected high- and middle-income countries (see Image 10.3). Poverty can be defined as living at less than 60% of the average (or median) income (Age UK, 2021). Practically speaking this means that a person does not have sufficient income to meet their basic needs or participate in society, including Internet access. Finance can therefore be a major barrier, with substantial numbers of older people around the world living in 'pensioner poverty'. With the massive shift of many services online facilitated by the COVID-19 pandemic, there are concerns that this has increased the digital divide among the socioeconomically disadvantaged, those in poor health, or socially isolated

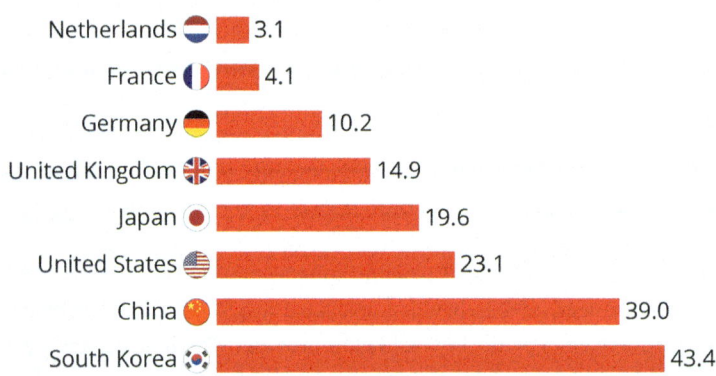

Image 10.3 OECD data on pensioner poverty. *Credit* Statista (www.statista.com)

(Heponiemi et al., 2020), i.e., those groups that the WHO believe can benefit most from remote delivery.

10.4.2 Accessibility and Usability of Equipment

A complicating factor with older adults is that their use of digital technology may be on a spectrum from non-users, drop-offs, intermittent users, and the fully connected. Some older adults are also self-excluders or 'digitally dismissive' (see Sect. 10.4.3). In a UK survey in 2022, more than half of those aged 70 or over (53%) did not use the Internet or have access to the Internet at home. The reasons given were 'don't need it', '[don't have the] skills', 'confidence', 'security', 'fraud' and 'costs' (Ofcom, 2022). Research has also found that the likelihood of using the Internet for essential services decreases with age. For example, in 2020, 76% of adults in the UK used the Internet for banking but this fell to 49% for those over 55 (ONS, 2019).

Some older adults feel that they cannot use technology to access services and may lack the skills to ensure they do so safely and not be open to scams, fraud, and viruses. It may be that utilising digital technologies is simply perceived as too complicated by older adults. Boyd and colleagues (2015) identified a lack of understanding of Facebook and a lack of perceived usefulness as the main barriers to older adults using it. In response, they created EasiSocial, a web application to display Facebook in a more user-friendly manner (Boyd et al., 2015). Following a 10-week training course, they found that EasiSocial was easier for older adults to use to access Facebook who were not frequent social network users.

Age-specific challenges to digital devices and services include physical alterations such as paralysis after a stroke, or tremors associated with Parkinson's disease, which may interfere with technology usage. The dexterity required to use new technologies is often highlighted as a problem, for example, smartphones are becoming increasingly popular for accessing the Internet, although some older people may prefer desktop computers, laptops and tablets for their form factor and larger screen sizes. Even older forms of technology using computer peripherals like a mouse, buttons or keys may be difficult to use for older adults (Damodaran et al., 2014). Poor eyesight is a particular problem when required to read small print or screens (McGrath & Astell, 2017). Other long-term health conditions may reduce people's energy, while chronic pain can interfere with concentration. Additionally, low mood may lower motivation to use digital resources, further exacerbating problems.

There is also a common lack of technology knowledge of what is available for older adults, where to access it, and how it could be beneficial. Many off-the-shelf technologies have functionality that could benefit older adults' everyday lives, but they often do not know what these are or how to find out about them.

10.4.3 Motivation, Support, and the 'Digitally Dismissive'

The term 'digitally excluded' may accurately be applied to those who have few opportunities to access AgeTech but want to learn and know about them. The term 'digitally dismissive' could be applied to those who do not want to learn or use these technologies at all (Plant et al., 2012). These technologies may be seen as a luxury for some, and unnecessary by others who have good social networks. Unfamiliarity with new ways of doing things and finding time to learn may make some older people more hesitant to invest their efforts and money.

People fear looking foolish if they cannot use a new device that they see others have mastered, and older people are no exception. They can also be insecure, or fearful of making mistakes or breaking an expensive device. Trust and confidence are major factors in using technologies, with negative attitudes and anxieties about scamming, viruses, and lack of privacy often seen among older adults. Previous experiences of using technology, the 'right' way of learning, and ongoing support are important to older people (Clayton et al., 2023). Although lack of interest is high on the list of reasons for not using the Internet, older adults will often ask someone else to get access for them (proxy users) most commonly to help buy something (Ofcom, 2022). Family and friends are the most common proxy users and the biggest sources of help in this context, using new technologies on behalf of older people. Without this support, digital exclusion is likely, which is exacerbated for isolated older adults.

10.5 Meeting the Exclusion Challenge

To maximise the use of AgeTech by older adults for Staying Connected, we need to challenge digital exclusion in all its forms. By supporting those who want to use AgeTech but currently do not (e.g. perhaps because of costs), providing support to increase confidence for those already using it (but who are not getting the most they can from it), and for those who may not want to use the technology (whether alternative services or access to a proxy user). The gap between those digitally included and excluded may eventually reduce as technology becomes increasingly ubiquitous but at present, there is still a need to address the digital divide. Policymakers, therefore, need to address issues of data poverty (access to the internet), device poverty (access to equipment) and skills poverty (the ability to use technology safely and with confidence) (Ofcom, 2022).

10.5.1 Addressing Data Poverty (Access to the Internet)

In response to the COVID-19 pandemic various national governments introduced initiatives to increase availability and access to the Internet which could be adopted or adapted elsewhere post-pandemic. The Connecting Families program, for example, was originally announced by the Canadian government in the 2017 budget to bring affordable Internet access to low-income families through the voluntary participation of Internet Service Providers. The second stage introduced in October 2021, expanded the program to include low-income seniors, giving them access to fast Internet speeds (50/10 megabits per second (Mbps)) for $20 per month. A similar program was announced in the US in November 2021 to bring the Internet to 48 million low-income households for $30 per month. Other initiatives include Pueblo Connect, an NSF-funded research project working with Native American Reservation communities in New Mexico to improve Internet access in economically marginalized communities and build local capacity for creating digital content.[2]

10.5.2 Addressing Device Poverty (Access to Equipment)

With free or affordable Internet, people will also need devices to access it. For people who cannot afford Internet access, devices are also likely to be inaccessible, including smartphones. Again, some initiatives exist which have tried to address this issue. In the United States, for example, older people can apply for a computer from Computers for Causes, a not-for-profit that makes donated computers available to low-income households including older people.[3] Information about other support available for low-income households in the US is available from the Get Government Grants website.[4] Of course, to benefit from this resource, older people and families in need, must first know of its existence and second have a way to access it.

During the pandemic several national governments launched a variety of programs get devices into low-income households, primarily to support continued access to education for children and young people during the lockdowns. This includes the Connecting Families program in Canada which partnered with Computers for Success Canada to provide computers to low-income Canadians. In the UK, the government provided more than 1.35 million laptops and tablets to schools and other education providers for disadvantaged children and young people to borrow. The scheme was supported by the 'Get Help With Technology' program, providing grants for schools to get support for setting up and resetting devices. This type of infrastructure support helped get devices into people's hands but also ensured they could use them, providing further examples of initiatives which could continue to make a difference post-pandemic.

---

[2] https://puebloconnect.cs.ucsb.edu.
[3] https://www.computerswithcauses.org/application/.
[4] https://getgovtgrants.com/.

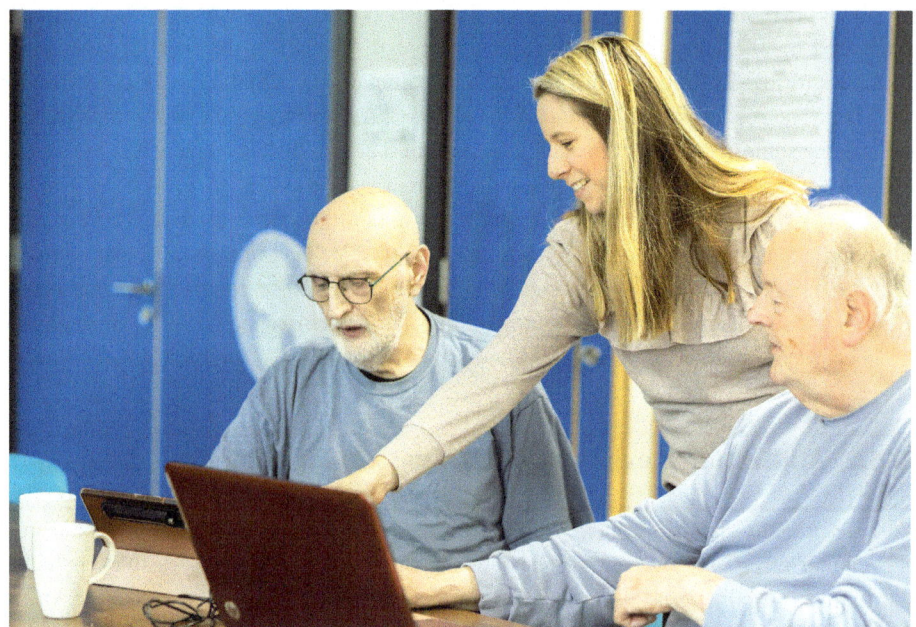

Image 10.4 *Credit* Independent age/ageing better

10.5.3 Addressing Skills Poverty (The Ability to Use Technology Safely and with Confidence)

Social connection through AgeTech is likely to be limited unless older adults are empowered to use it by developing digital skills and motivation. Initiatives to address digital skills have often focused on education, work and employment issues rather than the needs of an older adult to use digital technology for leisure and social connection (Image 10.4).

However, some learning can be taken from this approach. An example is Computers in Homes/Rorohiko I roto ngā KāInga, for low-income households in New Zealand. Families receive training in digital skills, a refurbished computer or smart device, 12 months of subsidised internet access and technical support for $50NZ. Computers in Homes is supported by funding from the New Zealand government to reach families through schools in low-income communities. Whilst not aimed at older people, this program provides a model that could be adopted for older adults.

Many initiatives that focus on older adults are found in the charity sector and highlight particular digital issues of concern for older adults like safety, relevance and the right support.[5] How an older adult is supported with digital technologies is likely to be

---

[5] For a useful guide see https://www.goodthingsfoundation.org/insights/doing-digital-in-later-life-a-practical-guide/.

important for their motivation ensuring that it is accessible and based on the needs of the individual. There are various examples of schemes to increase digital skills amongst older people including The Good Things Foundation 'Learn My Way'[6] and 'Make it Click'.[7] Skills can be learnt in various settings and to suit different learning styles. Examples include Digital Buddies,[8] where young volunteers are linked to an older adult to provide 1:1 support and Techmates,[9] a YouTube channel that provides online video support.

10.6 Not Just Assistive Technology

Another challenge for policymakers is to provide AgeTech devices which are not regarded as health or social care Assistive Technology. One reason that the provision of the Internet and computers or smart devices has been slow, is that they are consumer goods. Before the pandemic, these items were seen as luxuries but the requirement to shift to remote delivery of so many aspects of daily life transformed them into necessities. This breakthrough was required to shift thinking in policy beyond traditional definitions of Assistive Technology but there is still some way to go. In both insurance-based and free at the point of delivery healthcare systems, medical devices (e.g., blood glucose monitors) and assistive technologies (e.g., mobility aids) have undergone assessment and certification and so can be prescribed. Off the shelf, consumer goods will lack this assessment and certification and will pose a problem for healthcare and social care systems despite being vital to staying connected.

As demonstrated throughout this book, staying connected calls for the provision of devices as mandatory for mental, physical, and cognitive health. Much of the evidence demonstrating the importance of staying connected is preventive actions, for example, lowering the risk of dementia or depression. Whether prevention falls in the remit of healthcare or some other aspect of government is for policymakers to determine. However, one way to achieve this could be to extend definitions and certification of assistive technologies to include consumer goods. If devices for staying connected are included in an expanded health and social care provision, this could also bring the necessary infrastructure of training and support required to use them and address those aspects of the digital divide highlighted above.

---

[6] https://www.goodthingsfoundation.org/learn/learn-my-way/.

[7] https://www.goodthingsfoundation.org/insights/making-it-click-supporting-people-with-low-internet-use/.

[8] https://www.ageuk.org.uk/eastlondon/get-involved/volunteer/digital-buddies/.

[9] https://www.youtube.com/@TechMates/about.

10.7 The Technology Pipeline and Need for Co-creation, Co-design, and Co-production

Issues of digital exclusion for older adults are multi-dimensional. As highlighted above, there are multiple challenges to accessing and leveraging all of the potential benefits of AgeTech for staying connected. Implementation and adoption of new devices require constant training and support. Infrastructure must be put in place to establish truly connected societies that are flexible enough to keep up with new developments as they emerge. This is one of the 'wicked' problems of our times as commercial products constantly change to sell more devices. However, people on fixed incomes who are provided with reconditioned laptops or smart devices, do not have the opportunity to change these. Constant operating system upgrades currently make these devices obsolete after a certain amount of time. Policymakers, therefore, need to work with large technology companies to develop solutions that enable disadvantaged users to keep using their devices whilst allowing the companies to continue their core business.

Inclusive digital design also continues to be an issue and the involvement of older adults in creating digital services and products is essential to ensure they are successfully adopted by them. A more concerted effort is needed by technology companies to harness the involvement of older adults in the co-creation, co-design and co-production of AgeTech. For older users of technology, human need is likely to be of central concern for their use and so we must understand their experiences and attitudes. This requires much greater funding from policymakers for evidence gathering plus a move away from the traditional randomized controlled trial. This need was recognized at the end of the last century by Mowatt and colleagues (1997) who sought to identify factors that influenced health technology assessments of emerging medical devices. With commercially available products such as tablets or smartphones, the frequent operating system updates, which can subtly change the interface and modes of interaction with familiar apps, make large-scale RCTs over any substantial timeframe infeasible.

While computers and smart devices plus a multitude of accessible and useful apps already exist, many of the initiatives and devices considered in this book are prototypes that have not gone beyond the early development stage. Others, such as Hug Shirt have taken nearly 20 years to become available products. Closing the gap between promising ideas and products in people's hands, needs to be taken as seriously as drug development to create a comparable pipeline. We need to recognise digital technologies are no longer simply luxury items or expensive toys but are central to the social, economic, and political life of older adults. There is a need for policymakers to promote them as a 'social good' (Aarts et al., 2021) and address the digital inequalities that will reduce social connection and potentially lead to further loneliness and social isolation.

References

Aarts, E., Fleuren, H., Sitskoorn, M., & Wilthagen T. (2021). Internet access as an essential social good. *Nature Public Health Emergency Collection*, 29–33. https://doi.org/10.1007/978-3-030-65355-2_4

Age UK. (2021). Poverty in Later Life. Available at https://www.ageuk.org.uk/globalassets/age-uk/documents/policy-positions/money-atters/poverty_in_later_life_briefing_june_2021.pdf

Boyd, K., Nugent, C., Donnelly, M., Sterritt, R. et al. (2015). EasiSocial: An innovative way of increasing adoption of social media in older people. In C. Bodine, S. Helal, T. Gu & M. Mokhtari (Eds.), *Smart Homes and Health Telematics. ICOST 2014. Lecture Notes in Computer Science* (8456). Springer. https://doi.org/10.1007/978-3-319-14424-5_3

Clayton, D., de Vries, K., Clifton, A., Cousins, E. et al. (2023). "Like an unbridled horse that runs away with you": A study of older and disabled people during the COVID-19 pandemic and their use of digital technologies, *Disability and Society*, 1–23. https://doi.org/10.1080/09687599.2023.2217470

Damant, J., & Knapp, M. (2015). *What are the Likely Changes in Society and Technology Which Will Impact Upon the Ability of Older Adults to Maintain Social (Extra-Familial) Networks of Support Now, in 2025 and in 2040?* Government Office for Science.

Damodaran, L., Olphert, T. W., & Sandhu, J. (2014). Falling off the bandwagon? Exploring the challenges to sustained digital engagement by older people. *Gerontology, 60*(2), 163–173.

Heponiemi, T., Jormanainen, V., Leemann, L., Manderbacka, K., et al. (2020). Digital divide in perceived benefits of online health care and social welfare services: National cross-sectional survey study. *Journal of Medical Internet Research, 22*(7), e17616. https://doi.org/10.2196/17616

McGrath, C., & Astell, A. (2017). The benefits and barriers to technology acquisition: Understanding the decision-making processes of older adults with Age-Related Vision Loss (ARVL). *British Journal of Occupational Therapy, 80*(2), 123–131.

Mossberger, K., Tolbert, C. J., & Stansbury, M. (2003). *Virtual inequality: Beyond the digital divide.* Georgetown University Press.

Mowatt, G., Bower, D. J., Brebner, J. A., Cairns, J. A., et al. (1997). When and how to assess fast-changing technologies: A comparative study of medical applications of four generic technologies. *Health Technology Assessment, 1*(14), 1–149.

Ofcom (2022). *Digital Exclusion: A Review of Ofcom's Research on Digital Exclusion Among Adults in the UK*. Available at https://www.ofcom.org.uk/data/assets/pdf_file/0022/234364/digital-exclusion-review-2022.pdf

Older Adults Technology Services (OATS). Aging Connected (2021). Available at: https://agingconnected.org/report/

Office of National Statistics (ONS) (2019). Exploring the UK's Digital Divide. Available at: https://www.ons.gov.uk/peoplepopulationandcommunity/householdcharacteristics/homeinternetandsocialmediausage/articles/exploringtheuksdigitaldivide/2019-03-04

Plant, H., Aldridge, F., Bosley, S., Casey, L., et al. (2012). *Get digital: Impact study*. Niace.

Tsatsou, P. (2011). *Digital divides in Europe: Culture.* Peter Lang.

Yao, Y., Zhang, H., Liu, X., Liu, X., et al. (2021). Bridging the digital divide between old and young people in China: Challenges and opportunities. *The Lancet Healthy Longevity, 2*(3), 125–126.

Emerging Issues and Future Directions 11

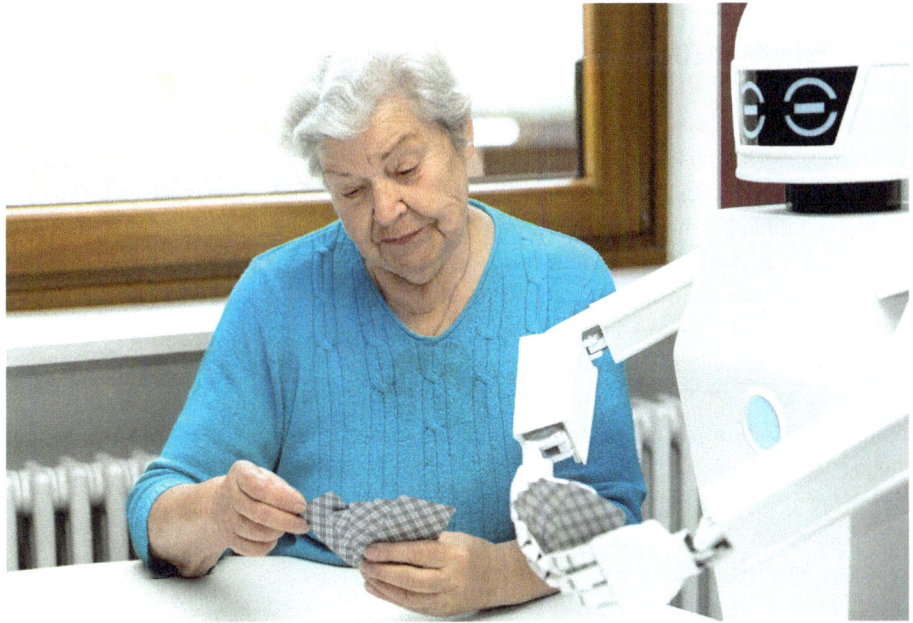

Image 11.1 *Credit* Shutterstock–Miriam Doerr Martin Frommherz

© The Author(s), under exclusive license to Springer Nature Switzerland AG 2026
A. Astell and D. Clayton, *AgeTech for Staying Connected*, Synthesis Lectures on
Technology and Health, https://doi.org/10.1007/978-3-031-87031-6_11

11.1 The Challenge

As demonstrated elsewhere in this book, the COVID-19 pandemic speeded up the introduction of technologies, particularly remote delivery of services across the world. Many aspects of this are positive in terms of upending pervasive negative perceptions about the willingness and interest of older adults in using technology (they are interested which researchers have known for many years) (Image 11.1). However, through necessity much of this rapid switch to digital was done with whatever was to hand, leveraging the knowledge or skills of staff from using their personal devices. There has been limited opportunity to develop infrastructure and make any medium to long-term plans. Now that the COVID-19 pandemic is past, there is plenty of opportunity to reflect on lessons learnt and how we can use these experiences for developing robust future services for aging well.

11.2 What's in This Chapter?

This chapter will explore some of these emerging issues for the application of AgeTech and offers some advice to service providers and practitioners to reflect upon when thinking about working with older adults to use AgeTech for social connection. Changes in society will be highlighted as how we should be careful to ethically incorporate technology into the lives of older adults and services to support and care for them. This is illustrated with a real-life example from healthcare. In a recent article about social isolation in a post-pandemic world, the authors highlighted the potential to see more, rather than less social isolation with the increased use of technology for social connection and support services (Clayton & Astell, 2022). A personalised approach for dealing with loneliness and social isolation is therefore put forward to urge service providers and practitioners interested in utilising technologies with older adults to also keep the more 'traditional' face-to-face options open. Men in Sheds, a non-technical innovation to address the specific problem of loneliness for older men is highlighted through the case study of Mr. Emeka who is isolated from social groups, community and family.

11.3 Older Age and Societal Change

Contemporary societies are very different from those that previous generations experienced. Victor et al. (2009) suggest that it is easy to overlook the magnitude of structural change and how these changes provide a new context within which old age and later life are experienced. They cite changes that included demographic change e.g. how people are living longer, reorganisation of work/leisure, the role of women, immigration, legislative change, rising levels of prosperity amongst the old, the impact of globalisation and global capitalism, and changes in social attitudes and norms towards aging.

We can add digital technological innovation to these structural changes which are aiding the transformation of social relationships (Nowland et al., 2018). Social relationships are not just shaped by individual characteristics or responses to life events, but also by these structural features of societies. Loneliness and social isolation can arguably be an indicator of the failure of contemporary societies to support social connections where the lonely get sicker and are more disadvantaged because they do not have people to take care of them or support them (Tomini et al., 2016). Traditional collective ways of life are replaced by individualism and self-reliance. In Japan, for example, the combination of an aging society and economic decline sees the rise in 'kodokushi'—people dying alone and remaining undiscovered for long periods.

11.4 Ethically Incorporating Technology into Services

Given economic and social pressures, technology is seen to offer the potential to address issues within the context of an environment of scarce resources e.g. staff shortages. However, there are some fears that the delivery of services by digital means will substitute real human contact rather than complementing and improving services for older adults. Healthcare has a long tradition of technology innovation and adoption for a wide range of activities. Frequently an early adopter of many technological developments, there are plenty of healthcare examples to draw on for developing our future models for service delivery. One example is the use of remote technology in healthcare. This presents complex questions regarding when and how it should be used, particularly when it is replacing face-to-face interactions. The following case from the United States highlights issues about the appropriateness and judgement in deciding to use technology over in-person visits.

11.4.1 Spotlight Issue—Telehealth for Delivering Bad News

Medical training is increasingly paying attention to delivering bad news to patients. Several frameworks have been developed across the world to deliver bad news, all based on face-to-face interviews. Collini et al. (2021) identified the following key factors for delivering bad news across settings and health conditions: 'ensuring privacy and adequate time without interruptions, clarity and honesty when delivering the information, and an empathetic and caring attitude' (p. 151). In March 2019 the 16-year-old granddaughter of a 79-year-old man with lung cancer recorded the visit between her grandfather and the doctor delivering the results of investigations that had been carried out into his shortness of breath. The doctor 'arrived' via a telepresence robot to tell the gentleman that there was not much more they could do but make him 'comfortable'.

The family posted this video,[1] which prompted questions about the appropriateness of using telepresence to deliver bad news and the more general incorporation of telemedicine into healthcare. In her Bill of Health (Petrie-Flom Centre, Harvard Law School) article examining this case, Adriana Krasniansky identifies that telemedicine can cut operating costs, increase access to care and potentially reduce physician burnout. The downside, she suggests, is…

> … the propensity to create even more emotional distance between a patient and doctor, especially if the two do not have an established rapport". (Krasniansky, 2019)

While this example took place in a hospital setting, the issues related to emotional distance and rapport are relevant to remote clinical interactions where patients are at home or in other settings.

11.4.2 Face-to-Face Versus Remote Contact

In the post-pandemic world, these ethical and practice issues remain important in decisions about the structure and the nature of a whole variety of services going forward. Although just one example, this shows the importance of considering how technology can, could and should be incorporated into personal, local, national, and global infrastructures to deliver the benefits of aging well. Concerns have also been raised that rather than promoting interaction telehealth, for example, can increase social isolation (Daborwska & Cornford, 1998). Specific concerns were identified by the UK Social Care Institute for Excellence 2010 report on the ethical issues in the use of telecare, relating to in-person visits being replaced by remote visits and passive monitoring of individuals in their homes (Perry et al., 2010).

For some older adults, anything other than face-to-face contact is likely to be insufficient. This was brought sharply into focus by the COVID-19 pandemic and enforced isolation of so many people across many months of 2020 and 2021, particularly older adults who were exposed to higher degrees of restrictions and isolation because of their vulnerability to the more serious outcomes associated with the virus (Dahlberg, 2021). Despite the surge in the use of video-calling services during this time (Burkitt-Gray, 2021), pre-pandemic evidence of the effectiveness of video calls in addressing social isolation in older adults was deemed uncertain (Noone et al., 2020). A study of inter-household contact in the US and the UK during the pandemic reported that more frequent

---

[1] The video recording posted by the family can be viewed here: https://blog.petrieflom.law.harvard.edu/2019/09/11/navigating-sensitive-hospital-conversations-in-the-age-of-telemedicine/.

virtual contact led to increased feelings of loneliness in the older adult population (Hu & Qian, 2021).

A key message is therefore to recognise that real personal human social contact remains very important to older adults (Image 11.2). Being able to hear, touch, be close to or just be in the presence of another person is often described as the most important aspect of interaction for them (Clayton, 2018). Therefore, whilst remote methods of delivering services and staying in contact may be one approach to tackling loneliness and social isolation in society, there should be a consideration for other devices, services and community initiatives that create opportunities for people who are socially isolated to make direct connections with others. This is illustrated below via the case of Mr. Emeka.

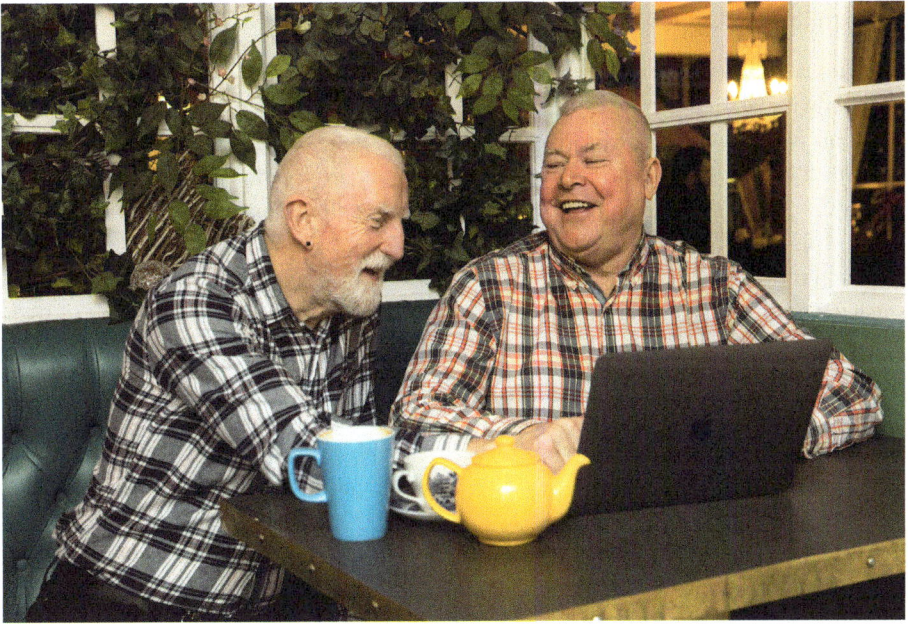

Image 11.2 *Credit* Independent age/ageing better

11.5 Persona and Scenario: Mr. Emeka[2]

Persona: Mr. Emeka is a 70-year-old man from the eastern part of Nigeria. He was a very wealthy businessman in his early life who travelled across many countries and barely had time for his family. He believed that all a man needs to do for his family is to support them financially. Most of his friends were his business partners, and he did not have any friends outside his business circle. He did not have close relationships with his two children because of his busy business schedules and travels. Nigeria adopts a collectivist culture that expects wealthy people (more financially comfortable than the average person) to help others within their wider community. However, Mr. Emeka was financially responsible for his nuclear family and did not help extended family members that much. Even though he financially provides for his family, no relationship was built between him and his children. As a result, he deprived himself of the opportunity to build meaningful relationships with family and friends in his early life.

Scenario: Mr. Emeka is now retired and was recently diagnosed with Glaucoma. He moved in with his first son, two grandchildren and his daughter-in-law for closer supervision of his health condition. Mr. Emeka had lost his ability to drive, and his son provided him with a driver that takes him to the pub (customarily called "beer parlour") every Saturday evening. Because he has not developed the skills of making friends in his early life, he struggled to connect with other older adults that also visit the pub. Also, his son stopped him from going to the pub for fear of neighbourhood insecurity and exposure to danger. Over time, his condition worsened, and he needed more care and desired to spend more time with his children and their families, but none of them could reciprocate. His children only provide him money for upkeep and rarely talk or have a conversation with him.

Mr. Emeka reported that even though he lives with his only son and family, he feels lonely as they hardly talk to him or even share a meal with him. Mr. Emeka stated that they exchange pleasantries, but there was no deep connection between him, his son, daughter-in-law, and grandchildren. He attributed this lack of deep connection to the weak relationship he had with his children throughout his life course; he only provided financial help and did not spend quality time with his children. Mr. Emeka described how lonely he is to his eye doctor, who referred him to a social worker that evaluated his case and referred him to a therapist. Mr. Emeka and his two children are currently working with a therapist to devise strategies to ensure that Mr. Emeka is feeling connected to his family. For instance, the therapist suggested that his other child and grandchildren not living with him could always make a conscious effort to keep close contact with their father through video and voice calls, as this will help create a reassurance of worth in their father.

---

[2] Persona and scenario created by Blessing U. Ojembe B.Sc., M.Sc., Ph.D.(c); Michael E. Kalu, BMR.PT, M.Sc., Ph.D.(c); and Oyinlola Oluwagbemiga, BSW, MSW of McMaster University, Canada.

11.5 Persona and Scenario: Mr. Emeka

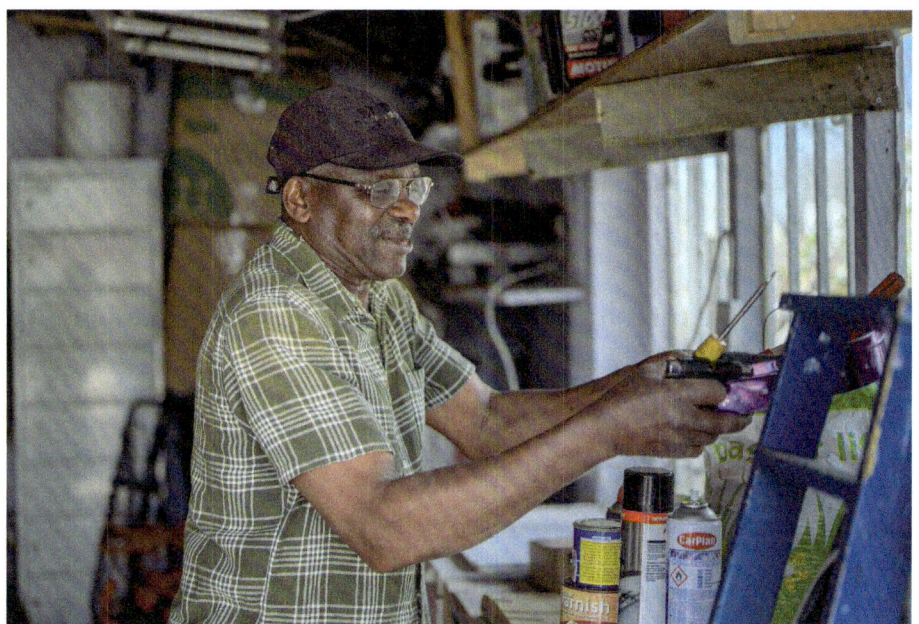

Image 11.3 *Credit* David Tett/ageing better

11.5.1 Spotlight on Community Initiatives: Men in Sheds

The case of Mr. Emeka is an emerging situation in Nigeria that draws attention to the wider issue of older men's experiences of loneliness and social isolation across the world (Beach & Bamford, 2014). A recent UK study identified '*social dislocation*' as a theme running through older men's experiences of loneliness and social isolation (Willis et al., 2020). This research, which included interviews with single and gay men living in urban and rural areas, some alone and some as caregivers for a partner, identified different ways in which older men experience loneliness. They identified a '*sense of social separation and estrangement*' from their communities and opportunities for making new relationships (Willis et al., 2020).

Men's Sheds are '*community spaces for men to connect, converse, and create*'.[3] Originating in Australia in the 1990s, Men's Sheds were developed to address a range of concerns about men's physical and mental health, and reluctance to seek help from traditional services (Waling & Fildes, 2017). Sheds are spaces for men to get together in person for activities such as woodworking, repairs, music, and watching TV (Image 11.3). They can help men to maintain friendship networks as well as improve how they feel about themselves, especially after leaving paid employment or being unemployed. Men's Sheds

---
[3] https://menssheds.org.uk/.

can be seen to provide safe spaces for men who are marginalized, reluctant or unable to access formal services, especially concerning health (Kelly et al., 2021). They are also suitable for those digitally excluded or digitally dismissive.

There are currently more than 600 Men's Sheds in the UK, with 150 more being planned. In the UK there are Men's Sheds Associations in each of the four home nations, England, Scotland, Wales and Northern Island. Other countries with Men's Sheds include Australia,[4] Canada,[5] New Zealand[6] and the United States.[7]

11.6 A Personalised Approach to Addressing Social Isolation and Loneliness

Supporting the use of technology to address the social isolation and loneliness of older adults means creating a different kind of relationship with them; one depending on the biography, history, and situation of the individual. Service providers and practitioners should avoid treating older adults as a homogeneous group which risks replicating negative or positive stereotypes of older age and providing 'one size fits all' solutions. Social contact, isolation and loneliness need to be contextualised concerning age, gender, sexuality, class and ethnic identities which shape social relationships and the social world of later life (Victor et al., 2009). We can see this with the persona of Mr Emeka. In his situation, a key factor is his lack of close relationships with his children. So-called '*disengaged fathers*' (Wall et al., 2007) are men who…

> …focus on the principles of the male breadwinner model and of gender-differentiated autonomy. Having a family and children is essential to male identity but it is linked here to the idea of the husband as [the] main provider and "head" of the family. Emphasis on gender differentiation and on the ideology of separate spheres is strong: the woman does all the housework and caring (supported by other women if necessary), the man has separate timetables, interests, and hobbies. (p. 111)

This 'traditional' model of family and household arrangements, where fathers spend little time developing relationships with their children, can lead to the situation Mr. Emeka finds himself in and provides the background for any solutions including Men in Sheds.

---

[4] Australia Men's Shed Association: https://mensshed.org.
[5] Canada Men's Sheds: https://menssheds.ca/about-mens-sheds/.
[6] Menz Shed New Zealand: https://menzshed.org.nz.
[7] United States Men's Sheds Association: https://usmenssheds.org.

11.6.1 Focus on Individuals Who Need Support the Most

The example of Mr. Emeka highlights that service providers and practitioners may wish to consider a range of technical and non-technical solutions to help with loneliness and social isolation. They may also target those groups most at risk of social isolation and loneliness but also excluded from using technology where technical solutions to promote social connection are desired. Specific focus could be given, for example, to those most disadvantaged and who lack natural support; more loneliness is found for members of minority groups, lesbian, gay and trans people, those living in deprived urban areas, and living in remote rural areas. Informal carers also report lower levels of well-being due to loneliness.

As highlighted by Mr. Emeka, older men may also be one of these groups. In the UK, for example, loneliness among older men is increasing because the population is growing faster than women. The number of older men living alone is projected to reach around 1.5 million by 2030, an increase of nearly 65% (Beach & Bamford, 2014). One of the major challenges in addressing loneliness in older men is reaching them. By the very nature of being disconnected, isolated older men are difficult to reach. Many are living alone and do not come into contact with services if their physical health is okay including support to access digital technology. Even when they do have health problems, they do not think that their feelings are something to share with the doctor or even of importance. Recommendations from the research highlight the importance of understanding the reluctance of many men to speak about their experience of loneliness and to seek help, the ways in which other aspects of identity e.g. sexuality, interact with age, and recognising the needs of individuals (Willis et al., 2019).

A starting point is to build trust and confidence with these marginalised groups. This support may be required to be more intensive and focused than is currently being delivered by many service providers and will also need to include levels of financial support or benefits to enable engagement with AgeTech to purchase equipment and Internet services if desired.

11.6.2 Focus on Individual Outcomes with AgeTech

There is not a single experience or reality of social isolation and loneliness but rather a plurality of experiences. Thus, when considering if AgeTech could make a difference we need to understand these experiences. When considering the population level statistics, it could be easy to overlook the personal lived experience of social isolation and loneliness. A recent study identified five ways older people experience loneliness: feelings of loss or sadness triggered in the moment; changes in identity; loss of intimacy and grief/bereavement; reduced choice and control; and poor health and disadvantage (Clayton, 2018). This research also considers three strategies with which technology could be used to alleviate the different modes of loneliness: facilitating connections with other people; offering distraction from negative feelings; and enabling participation in therapeutic interventions.

In this context service providers and practitioners may wish to consider the outcomes AgeTech can bring for older adults who are lonely and socially isolated. This begins by assessing how technologies may help the older person through a detailed consideration of their loneliness experience, their preferred use and previous experiences of technology (and the support they have) and how using different technologies may help or not with social connectivity. It is an approach that involves person-centred thinking where different technologies are identified alongside different strategies for using these technologies. The overall aim is to find technological solutions that can meet the outcomes individuals want to achieve and will alleviate their loneliness and/or increase social contact. Some solutions have been highlighted in the different chapters of this book and can facilitate these conversations with older adults.

The discussion contained in this chapter has highlighted the potential for technology to both help and harm social connectivity. For some older adults technologies can encroach on the time they spend with other people, and they may fear that as more social interaction moves online, there will be fewer opportunities for them to have personal face-to-face contact which they prefer. Service providers, therefore, need to recognise technologies will not help everyone in the same way and some older adults will always require face-to-face interaction to achieve positive outcomes and stay connected.

References

Beach, B., & Bamford, S. M. (2014). Isolation: The Emerging Crisis for Older Men. A Report Exploring Experiences of Social Isolation and Loneliness Among Older Men in England. London, UK. Independent Age. Available at: https://www.independentage.org/policy-research/research-reports/isolation-emerging-crisis-for-older-men

Burkitt-Gray, A. (2021). 1.8bn People Using Mobile Video Calling After Covid Causes 50% growth. Available at:Chttps://www.capacitymedia.com/articles/3827719/18bn-people-using-mobile-video-calling-after-covid-causes-50-growth

Clayton, D. (2018). Exploring Loneliness Among Older People and Their Related Use of New Technologies. PhD thesis, University of Sheffield. http://etheses.whiterose.ac.uk

Clayton, D., & Astell, A. (2022). Social isolation and the role of AgeTech in a post-COVID world. *Healthcare Management Forum, 35*(5), 291–295.

Collini, A., Parker, H., & Oliver, A. (2021). Training for difficult conversations and breaking bad news over the phone in the emergency department. *Emergency Medicine Journal, 38*(2), 151–154.

Dabrowska, E., & Cornford, T. (1998). Policy and telehealth: Social implications of telehealth and telecare technologies. *AMCIS 1998 Proceedings, 20.* https://aisel.aisnet.org/amcis1998/20

Dahlberg, L. (2021). Loneliness during the COVID-19 pandemic. *Aging and Mental Health, 25*(7), 1161–1164. https://doi.org/10.1080/13607863.2021.1875195

Hu, Y., & Qian, Y. (2021). COVID-19, inter-household contact and mental well-being among older adults in the US and the UK. *Frontiers in Sociology, 6*(143), 1–15. https://doi.org/10.3389/fsoc.2021.714626

Kelly, D., Steiner, A., Mason, H., & Teasdale, S. (2021). Men's sheds as an alternative healthcare route? A qualitative study of the impact of Men's sheds on user's health improvement behaviours. *BMC Public Health, 21*, 553. https://doi.org/10.1186/s12889-021-10585-3

Krasniansky, A. (2019). Navigating Sensitive Hospital Conversations in the Age of Telemedicine. The Petrie-Flom Center. Harvard Law School. September 11. Available at:https://petrieflom.law.harvard.edu/2019/09/11/navigating-sensitive-hospital-conversations-in-the-age-of-telemedicine/

Noone, C., McSharry, J., Smalle, M., Burns, A., et al. (2020). Video calls for reducing social isolation and loneliness in older people: A rapid review. *Cochrane Database of Systematic Reviews, 5*(5), 1–40. https://doi.org/10.1002/14651858.CD013632

Nowland, R., Necka, E. A., & Cacioppo, J. T. (2018). Loneliness and social Internet use: Pathways to reconnection in a digital world? *Perspectives on Psychological Science, 13*(1), 70–87.

Perry, A. G., Moore, K. M., Levesque, L. E., Pickett, C. W., et al. (2010). A comparison of methods for forecasting emergency department visits for respiratory illness using telehealth Ontario calls. *Canadian Journal of Public Health, 101*(6), 464–469. https://doi.org/10.1007/BF03403965

Tomini, F., Tomini, S. M., & Groot, W. (2016). Understanding the value of social networks in life satisfaction of elderly people: A comparative study of 16 European countries using SHARE data. *BMC Geriatrics, 16*, 203. https://doi.org/10.1186/s12877-016-0362-7

Victor, C., Scambler, S., & Bond, J. (2009). *The Social World of Older People: Understanding Loneliness and Social Isolation in Later Life: Understanding loneliness and social isolation in later life*. McGraw-Hill Education.

Waling, A., & Fildes, D. (2017). 'Don't fix what ain't broke': Evaluating the effectiveness of a Men's Shed in inner-regional Australia. *Health and Social Care in the Community, 25*(2), 758–768.

Wall, K., Aboim, S., & Marinho, S. (2007). Fatherhood, family and work in men's lives: Negotiating new and old masculinities. *Recherches Sociologiques Et Anthropologiques, 38*(2), 105–122. https://doi.org/10.4000/rsa.470

Willis, P., Vickery, A., Hammond, J., Symonds, J., Jessiman, T., & Abbott, D. (2019). Addressing older men's experiences of loneliness and social isolation in later life. Policy Report, April 2019, University of Bristol. Available at: http://www.bristol.ac.uk/media-library/sites/policybristol/PolicyBristol-PolicyReport-51-Apr2019-OMAM.pdf

Willis, P., Vickery, A., & Jessiman, T. (2020). Loneliness, social dislocation, and invisibility experienced by older men who are single or living alone: Accounting for differences across sexual identity and social context. *Ageing and Society, 42*(2), 409–431.

Conclusion

12

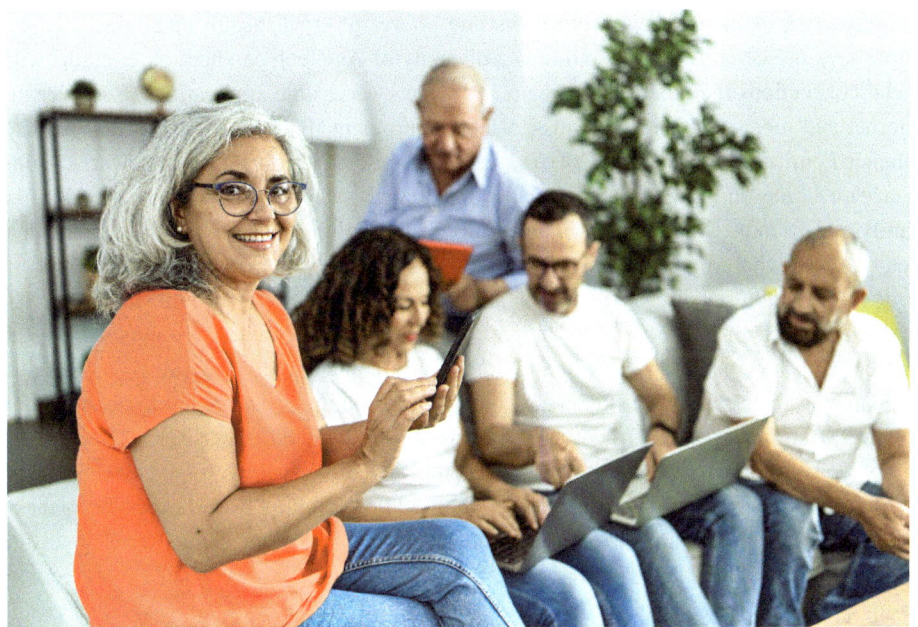

Image 12.1 *Credit* Shutterstock–Krakenimages.com

This book has explored the multiple ways in which staying connected is vital for human health and well-being and how AgeTech may provide solutions to support older people (Image 12.1). We have seen in Chapter Two how loneliness and social isolation are multidimensional and complex issues, and how staying connected is an important aspect of tackling these issues. The scenario from Mrs. Adeniyi highlighted that multiple factors can lead to older adults becoming lonely and isolated potentially leading to poor health and quality of life outcomes. Whether or not loneliness in the older generations is an 'epidemic' is open to debate (Berg-Weger & Morley, 2020; Ortiz-Ospina, 2019), stemming largely again from the distinction between loneliness and social isolation, but its presence within society is unquestionable. A review of survey data from 15 countries over the last decade reveals between 25 and 62% of older adults self-reporting some degree of loneliness (Ortiz-Ospina & Roser, 2020). The majority of the countries featured in this survey are Western European, as well as the US and Israel, but figures falling within this range or higher have also been reported in China (Luo & Waite, 2014), Brazil (Torres et al., 2021), Uganda (Nzabona et al., 2016), and Australia (Ogrin et al., 2021), indicating that it is a global issue.

Social interaction is fundamental to human existence from birth, situating us as social beings in a social world. Lack of social interaction can lead to feelings of loneliness, increased risk of mental health problems and poorer physical health outcomes. Chapter Three saw the scenario of Wen and how a diversity of AgeTech can help older adults with social connections including mainstream and widely accessible applications used over the Internet and more sophisticated and specialist equipment like robots and Virtual Reality. Chapter Four provided examples of AgeTech that might support those, like Maria, living in a care home and wanting to stay in contact with her existing social networks like family and friends. This includes innovations like teledining. The focus of Chapter Five was on those who are socially isolated with few social contacts. Through the scenario of Simon, we could see how AgeTech such as chatbots and mood apps would support mental health and bereavement difficulties and potentially support those who are most isolated to connect with new people by facilitating community contact and befriending.

Engaging in activities with others such as dancing, singing, and going to concerts and galleries, also provides enjoyment and pleasure which we need in our lives. The focus of Chapter Six was on how AgeTech is increasingly enabling access to social and leisure activities for older adults. The scenario of Mathilda highlighted how the development of innovations like online art, virtual tours and gaming enable older adults to enjoy leisure even when socially isolated and lonely. Some of these activities benefit from remote groups like singing and music making, while others are solitary activities but enable those alone to undertake a meaningful and enjoyable activity to take them away from their isolation.

Social interaction can also contribute to cognitive health, with benefits shown in reducing dementia risk. Chapter Seven deals with this important issue and through the example of Susan, we see how Age Tech can be used like games and dancing to promote physical and social activities that will support those with cognitive impairment to stay social, active and healthy for longer. Digital Innovations also include those which enable older adults to tell and recount their stories. Chapter Eight moved on to discuss the sensitive issues of intimacy. We need intimate connections with others through hugs, touch, or sexual activity. For older adults, loss of intimacy is often the result of bereavement and although AgeTech may not be able to replace human interaction it can be used to facilitate intimate encounters and even substitute for human touch. Through the example of Edwin, we saw different aspects explored for using AgeTech to simulate intimacy and innovations like dating apps and online sexual activity that may support others to find real intimacy. Chapter Nine highlights the importance of staying connected and healthcare. As we age, we are more likely to need healthcare treatment and/or advice, about how to stay healthy including support to change behaviours which could benefit us. The scenario of Mei highlights how Age Tech can provide self-management tools like chatbots and telecare to deliver healthcare interventions, promote education and peer support about conditions online and over distances and support positive aging.

In examining these topics above, the book has explored the wide variety of technology, applications, and services available or in development for helping older adults stay connected in later life. Technology, however, does not exist in a vacuum. To realise the benefits and empower people to live and age as well as possible, access to the Internet has to be seen as a human right, with support and access to devices for everyone. Chapter Ten discusses the digital divide and what policy needs to address. To stay connected, individuals must have people or things, e.g., services, and activities, to be connected with. To be of use, technology has to be incorporated into people's lives. This requires it to be available, accessible, and affordable either to individuals or for services to provide. Individuals need to be aware of what technologies are available and they need opportunities to try technologies, to see if they will deliver benefits and fit into their lives.

Changes in digital technologies have seen them spread globally, grow rapidly, change in nature, and at a pace that few could predict. Services need to plan how to implement technologies, and how to add them in ways that benefit their users or clients, their staff, and their operations. These ethical issues require understanding and are briefly touched upon above along with a call to consider a personalised approach to the way that promotes the use of technologies to help with social connection. The pandemic has changed forever our ideas about remote service delivery and the role of AgeTech in people's lives. We need to be mindful of both the help and harm it adds to social connection and by doing so, make older adults feel optimistic and in touch with the world.

References

Berg-Weger, M. and Morley, J.E. (2020) Loneliness in Old Age: An Unaddressed Health Problem. Journal of Nutrition, Health and Aging 24, 243–245 (2020). https://doi.org/10.1007/s12603-020-1323-6

Luo, Y., & Waite, L. J. (2014). Loneliness and mortality among older adults in China. *Journals of Gerontology—Series B Psychological Sciences and Social Sciences, 69*(4), 633–645. https://doi.org/10.1093/geronb/gbu007

Nzabona, A., Ntozi, J., & Rutaremwa, G. (2016). Loneliness among older persons in Uganda: Examining social, economic, and demographic risk factors. *Ageing and Society, 36*(4), 860–888. https://doi.org/10.1017/S0144686X15000112

Ogrin, R., Cyarto, E. V., Harrington, K. D., Haslam, C., Lim, M. H., et al. (2021). Loneliness in older age: What is it, why is it happening, and what should we do about it in Australia?. *Australasian Journal on Ageing, 40*(2), 202–207.

Ortiz-Ospina, E. (2019). "Is there a loneliness epidemic?" Published online at OurWorldinData.org. Retrieved from: https://ourworldindata.org/loneliness-epidemic'.

Ortiz-Ospina, E., & Roser, M. (2020). Loneliness and Social Connections. OurWorldinData.org. Available at: https://ourworldindata.org/social-connections-and-loneliness

Torres, J. L., de Braga, L., S., Moreira, B. de S., Sabino Castro, C. M., et al. (2021). Loneliness and social disconnectedness in the time of pandemic period among Brazilians: Evidence from the ELSI COVID-19 initiative. *Aging and Mental Health, 26*(5), 898–904. https://doi.org/10.1080/13607863.2021.1913479

The manufacturer's authorised representative in the EU is Springer Nature Customer Service Centre GmbH, Europaplatz 3, 69115 Heidelberg, Germany. If you have any concerns regarding our products, please contact ProductSafety@springernature.com

Printed and bound by CPI Group (UK) Ltd, Croydon, CR0 4YY

18/02/2026

02055607-0002